PET Imaging in Melanoma

Guest Editors

DAVID FUSTER, MD, PhD
DOMENICO RUBELLO, MD

PET CLINICS

www.pet.theclinics.com

Consulting Editor
ABASS ALAVI, MD, PhD (Hon), DSc (Hon)

January 2011 • Volume 6 • Number 1

SAUNDERS an imprint of ELSEVIER, Inc.

W.B. SAUNDERS COMPANY
A Division of Elsevier Inc.

1600 John F. Kennedy Boulevard • Suite 1800 • Philadelphia, Pennsylvania 19103-2899

http://www.theclinics.com

PET CLINICS Volume 6, Number 1
January 2011 ISSN 1556-8598, ISBN-13: 978-1-4557-0488-0

Editor: Barton Dudlick
Developmental Editor: Jessica Demetriou

PET Clinics (ISSN 1556-8598) is published quarterly by Elsevier Inc., 360 Park Avenue South, New York, NY 10010-1710. Months of issue are January, April, July, and October. Periodicals postage paid at New York, NY, and additional mailing offices. Subscription prices per year are $199.00 (US individuals), $279.00 (US institutions), $102.00 (US students), $226.00 (Canadian individuals), $312.00 (Canadian institutions), $124.00 (Canadian students), $241.00 (foreign individuals), $312.00 (foreign institutions), and $124.00 (foreign students). To receive student and resident rate, orders must be accompanied by name of affiliated institution, date of term, and the signature of program/residency coordinator on institution letterhead. Orders will be billed at individual rate until proof of status is received. Foreign air speed delivery is included in all Clinics subscription prices. All prices are subject to change without notice. POSTMASTER: Send address changes to PET Clinics, Elsevier Health Sciences Division, Subscription Customer Service, 3251 Riverport Lane, Maryland Heights, MO 63043. **Customer Service: 1-800-654-2452 (U.S. and Canada); 314-447-8871 (outside U.S. and Canada). Fax: 314-447-8029. E-mail: journalscustomerservice-usa@elsevier.com (for print support); journalsonlinesupport-usa@elsevier.com (for online support).**

Reprints. For copies of 100 or more of articles in this publication, please contact the Commercial Reprints Department, Elsevier Inc., 360 Park Avenue South, New York, NY 10010-1710. Tel.: 212-633-3812; Fax: 212-462-1935; E-mail: reprints@elsevier.com.

Printed and bound in the United Kingdom
Transferred to Digital Print 2011

Contributors

CONSULTING EDITOR

ABASS ALAVI, MD, PhD(Hon), DSc(Hon)
Professor of Radiology, Division of Nuclear
Medicine, University of Pennsylvania School of
Medicine, Philadelphia, Pennsylvania

GUEST EDITORS

DAVID FUSTER, MD, PhD
Nuclear Medicine Department, Hospital Clínic,
University of Barcelona, Barcelona, Spain

DOMENICO RUBELLO, MD
Professor, Department of Nuclear Medicine,
PET Center, Santa Maria della Misericordia
Hospital, Rovigo, Italy

AUTHORS

ABASS ALAVI, MD, PhD(Hon), DSc(Hon)
Professor of Radiology, Division of Nuclear
Medicine, University of Pennsylvania
School of Medicine, Philadelphia,
Pennsylvania

ADIL AL-NAHHAS, FRCP
Professor, Department of Nuclear Medicine,
Imperial College Healthcare Trust,
Hammersmith Hospital, London,
United Kingdom

SORAYA BANAYAN, MD
Nuclear Medicine Physician, Saint-Louis
Hospital, University of Paris VII, Paris, France

BRIAN J. CZERNIECKI, MD
Assistant Professor of Surgery, Division of
Endocrine and Oncologic Surgery, Department
of Surgery, University of Pennsylvania School
of Medicine, Philadelphia, Pennsylvania

STEFANO FANTI, MD
UO Medicina Nucleare, Azienda Ospedaliero
Universitaria di Bologna Policlinico
S.Orsola-Malpighi, Bologna, Italy

DAVID FUSTER, MD, PhD
Nuclear Medicine Department, Hospital Clínic,
University of Barcelona, Barcelona, Spain

GAIA GRASSETTO, MD
Department of Nuclear Medicine,
PET Center, Santa Maria della Misericordia
Hospital, Rovigo, Italy

DAVID GROHEUX, MD
Nuclear Medicine Physician, Saint-Louis
Hospital, University of Paris VII,
Paris, France

BRIAN NG CHENG HIN, MBBS
Department of Nuclear Medicine, Imperial
College Healthcare Trust, Hammersmith
Hospital, London, United Kingdom

ELIF HINDIÉ, MD, PhD
Associate Professor of Nuclear Medicine,
Saint-Louis Hospital, University of Paris VII,
Paris, France

GIORGOS C. KARAKOUSIS, MD
Assistant Professor of Surgery, Division of
Endocrine and Oncologic Surgery, Department
of Surgery, University of Pennsylvania School
of Medicine, Philadelphia, Pennsylvania

SAMEER KHAN, FRCR
Department of Nuclear Medicine, Imperial
College Healthcare Trust, Hammersmith
Hospital, London, United Kingdom

CÉLESTE LEBBÉ, MD, PhD
Professor, Department of Dermatology,
Saint-Louis Hospital, Paris, France

JUSTIN E. MACKEY, MD
Fellow in the Department of Radiology,
Division of Body Imaging, Hospital of the
University of Pennsylvania, Philadelphia,
Pennsylvania

WING YAN MOK, MBBS
Department of Nuclear Medicine, Imperial
College Healthcare Trust, Hammersmith
Hospital, London, United Kingdom

JEAN-LUC MORETTI, MD, PhD
Professor, Nuclear Medicine, Saint-Louis
Hospital, University of Paris VII, Paris, France

CRISTINA NANNI, MD
UO Medicina Nucleare, Azienda Ospedaliero
Universitaria di Bologna Policlinico
S.Orsola-Malpighi, Bologna, Italy

FRANCESCA PONS, MD, PhD, FEBNM
Professor of Medicine and Head,
Department of Nuclear Medicine,
Hospital Clínic, University of Barcelona;
Institut d'Investigacions Biomèdiques
August Pi Sunyer (IDIBAPS); Nuclear
Medicine Department CRC-MAR
Corporació Sanitària, Barcelona, Spain

DOMENICO RUBELLO, MD
Professor, Department of Nuclear Medicine,
PET Center, Santa Maria della Misericordia
Hospital, Rovigo, Italy

FARID SARANDI, MD
Nuclear Medicine Physician, Saint-Louis
Hospital, University of Paris VII,
Paris, France

DREW A. TORIGIAN, MD, MA
Assistant Professor of Radiology,
Department of Radiology, Hospital of the
University of Pennsylvania, University
of Pennsylvania School of Medicine,
Philadelphia, Pennsylvania

MARIE-ELISABETH TOUBERT, MD
Nuclear Medicine Physician, Saint-Louis
Hospital, University of Paris VII,
Paris, France

LAETITIA VERCELLINO, MD
Nuclear Medicine Physician, Saint-Louis
Hospital, University of Paris VII,
Paris, France

SERGI VIDAL-SICART, MD, PhD, FEBNM
Department of Nuclear Medicine, Hospital
Clínic, University of Barcelona; Institut
d'Investigacions Biomèdiques August Pi
Sunyer (IDIBAPS); Nuclear Medicine
Department, CRC-MAR Corporació
Sanitària, Barcelona, Spain

IMENE ZERIZER, FRCR
Department of Nuclear Medicine,
Imperial College Healthcare Trust,
Hammersmith Hospital, London,
United Kingdom

Contents

When cutaneous melanoma recurrence is suspected, several imaging techniques can be used to confirm or rule out this possibility as well as performing an adequate follow-up of the disease. [18F]Fluorodeoxyglucose (FDG)-PET may play an important role in this setting. Ultrasonography and FDG-PET can be useful in the assessment of regional node involvement but sentinel node biopsy is the gold standard. PET/computed tomography is most useful for identifying all metastatic sites before embarking on a metastasectomy of an apparently isolated lesion or for clarifying the nature of a suspicious lesion identified by CT scan.

Because no effective cures are available for cutaneous malignant melanoma, early diagnosis and accurate staging are of the utmost importance in increasing patient survival. Fluorodeoxyglucose positron emission tomography (PET)/computed tomography is a functional imaging technique that has contributed to ameliorating surveillance of patients with melanoma. New PET probes are under evaluation, and many have been tried in in vivo imaging protocols based on the use of small animal PET and animal models of cutaneous melanoma. Those compounds are targeted to a-melanocyte-stimulating hormone receptor and to the intracellular biosynthesis of melanin, and all of them showed promising results.

Noncutaneous melanoma is a rare entity for which there is still no agreement about management. The rarity of this disease has resulted in a lack of significant investigation and insufficient opportunity to evaluate the epidemiologic features, risk factors, and the most useful diagnostic and therapeutic approaches. Noncutaneous melanomas are characterized by poor prognosis, and the diagnosis is usually delayed because of their unusual locations and lack of physician awareness. This review focuses principally on ocular melanoma, the most frequent noncutaneous melanoma, for which each aspect of the disease is described. The potential utility of nuclear medicine procedures is also considered.

18F FDG-PET has proven its use as a technique in the field of melanoma, but there are valid concerns related to the specificity of 18F FDG-PET findings and the degree of accuracy we can expect in the assessment of response to new treatment protocols. The main avenues currently being explored for future use in staging and management of melanoma with PET other than FDG include monoclonal antibodies against melanoma-associated antigens, α-MSH analogues, amino acids involved in melanin formation, nicotinamide-based compounds, heterodimeric glycoproteins such as integrins, reporter gene imaging, cell proliferation, and hypoxia tracers.

PET Clinics

THE CLINICS ARE NOW AVAILABLE ONLINE!

Access your subscription at:
www.theclinics.com

GOAL STATEMENT
The goal of the *PET Clinics* is to keep practicing radiologists and radiology residents up to date with current clinical practice in positron emission tomography by providing timely articles reviewing the state of the art in patient care.

ACCREDITATION
PET Clinics is planned and implemented in accordance with the Essential Areas and Policies of the Accreditation Council for Continuing Medical Education (ACCME) through the joint sponsorship of the University of Virginia School of Medicine and Elsevier. The University of Virginia School of Medicine is accredited by the ACCME to provide continuing medical education for physicians.

The University of Virginia School of Medicine designates this educational activity for a maximum of 15 *AMA PRA Category 1 Credits*™ for each issue, 60 credits per year. Physicians should only claim credit commensurate with the extent of their participation in the activity.

The American Medical Association has determined that physicians not licensed in the US who participate in this CME activity are eligible for a maximum of 15 *AMA PRA Category 1 Credits*™ for each issue, 60 credits per year.

Category 1 credit can be earned by reading the text material, taking the CME examination online at http://www.theclinics.com/home/cme, and completing the evaluation. After taking the test, you will be required to review any and all incorrect answers. Following completion of the test and evaluation, your credit will be awarded and you may print your certificate.

FACULTY DISCLOSURE/CONFLICT OF INTEREST
The University of Virginia School of Medicine, as an ACCME accredited provider, endorses and strives to comply with the Accreditation Council for Continuing Medical Education (ACCME) Standards of Commercial Support, Commonwealth of Virginia statutes, University of Virginia policies and procedures, and associated federal and private regulations and guidelines on the need for disclosure and monitoring of proprietary and financial interests that may affect the scientific integrity and balance of content delivered in continuing medical education activities under our auspices.

The University of Virginia School of Medicine requires that all CME activities accredited through this institution be developed independently and be scientifically rigorous, balanced and objective in the presentation/discussion of its content, theories and practices.

All authors/editors participating in an accredited CME activity are expected to disclose to the readers relevant financial relationships with commercial entities occurring within the past 12 months (such as grants or research support, employee, consultant, stock holder, member of speakers bureau, etc.). The University of Virginia School of Medicine will employ appropriate mechanisms to resolve potential conflicts of interest to maintain the standards of fair and balanced education to the reader. Questions about specific strategies can be directed to the Office of Continuing Medical Education, University of Virginia School of Medicine, Charlottesville, Virginia.

The faculty and staff of the University of Virginia Office of Continuing Medical Education have no financial affiliations to disclose.

The authors/editors listed below have identified no professional or financial affiliations for themselves or their spouse/partner:
Abass Alavi, MD, PhD(Hon), DSc(Hon) (Consulting Editor); Adil Al-Nahhas, FRCP; Soraya Banayan, MD; Brian Ng Cheng Hin, MBBS; Brian J. Czerniecki, MD; Barton Dudlick (Acquisitions Editor); Stefano Fanti, MD; David Fuster, MD, PhD (Guest Editor); Gaia Grassetto, MD; David Groheux, MD; Elif Hindié, MD, PhD; Giorgos C. Karakousis, MD; Sameer Khan, FRCR; Céleste Lebbé, MD, PhD; Justin E. Mackey, MD; Wing Yan Mok, MBBS; Jean-Luc Moretti, MD, PhD; Cristina Nanni, MD; Francesca Pons, MD, PhD; Patrice Rehm, MD (Test Author); Domenico Rubello, MD (Guest Editor); Farid Sarandi, MD; Marie-Elisabeth Toubert, MD; Laetitia Vercellion, MD; Sergi Vidal-Sicart, MD, PhD; and Imene Zerizer, FRCR.

The authors/editors listed below identified the following professional or financial affiliations for themselves or their spouse/partner:
Drew A. Torigian, MD, MA is an industry funded research/investigator for Pfizer Corporation.

Disclosure of Discussion of Non-FDA Approved Uses for Pharmaceutical Products and/or Medical Devices.
The University of Virginia School of Medicine, as an ACCME provider, requires that all faculty presenters identify and disclose any off-label uses for pharmaceutical and medical device products. The University of Virginia School of Medicine recommends that each physician fully review all the available data on new products or procedures prior to clinical use.

TO ENROLL
To enroll in the PET Clinics Continuing Medical Education program, call customer service at 1-800-654-2452 or visit us online at www.theclinics.com/home/cme. The CME program is available to subscribers for an additional fee of $196.00.

Preface
PET Imaging in Melanoma

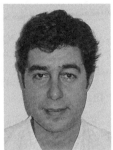 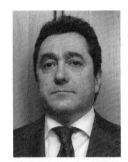

David Fuster, MD, PhD   Domenico Rubello, MD
Guest Editors

The incidence of malignant melanoma is increasing year by year, and despite a progressive improvement in overall survival rates, it is still a lethal cancer and an important cause of mortality. Melanoma is a very aggressive tumor, and prognosis depends mainly on the extent of the disease. If the tumor is diagnosed and treated at an early stage, the chances of survival are much higher. Prevention measures mainly focus on reducing the amount of sun exposure. Surveillance of pigmented skin lesions for early detection of suspected malignant melanoma is the means of controlling this tumor. A complete surgical resection with wide margins, depending on tumor thickness, is the elected treatment, but this is only effective in the early stages of the disease. Due to the higher risk of occult lymph node involvement, the American Joint Committee on Cancer has recommended the performance of sentinel lymph node biopsy in early-stage patients who present with invasive melanoma >1 mm in thickness with no clinically detectable nodal involvement or in 0.76- to 1-mm-thick lesions that are either ulcerated or have a high mitotic rate.

Early diagnosis of melanoma may occasionally be difficult, especially in those patients with lesions situated in atypical locations (the most frequent noncutaneous site being ocular melanoma), or in patients presenting with aggressive growth patterns or a rapid spread of disease. In such cases, surgery alone, with or without sentinel lymph node biopsy, may not be enough. Currently there is great need for further studies to investigate ways to improve staging and therapy of the disease. Anatomic and functional imaging techniques are useful and complementary in patients with melanoma. But when evaluating the possibility of locoregional melanoma spread or the presence of distant metastases, the most commonly used anatomic imaging procedures, namely x-ray, computed tomography, magnetic resonance, and ultrasound, are sometimes limited. Combined PET/CT is widely used, with promising results, especially in cases of advanced stage, suspected recurrence, and restaging of the disease prior to curative surgical intervention. However, for many aspects of the disease, such as initial diagnosis, or the staging of melanoma in early stages or the assessment of therapeutic response, the role of PET/CT has yet to be clearly established.

New PET probes that are selective for melanoma cells are currently being evaluated, and several in vivo imaging protocols, based on the use of small animal PET, have been attempted with promising, albeit preliminary results. Recent studies are starting to investigate the potential role of other

PET Clin 6 (2011) ix–x
doi:10.1016/j.cpet.2011.03.001
1556-8598/11/$ – see front matter

radiotracers to achieve greater specificity in diagnosis, characterization, staging, and treatment protocols of melanoma. Both preclinical studies using animal models and the introduction of radiotracers that are more specific than FDG will need to be developed in coming years in order to better understand and treat patients with melanoma.

In the articles that follow, all these issues will be thoroughly explored and analyzed by experts in the field, with the aim of determining where and when PET/CT can be of most help in the management of malignant melanoma. The latest trends in research, focusing on animal models, and the development of newer, more effective radiotracers, are also evaluated in depth.

David Fuster, MD, PhD
Nuclear Medicine Department
Hospital Clínic of Barcelona
Villarroel, 170
08036 Barcelona, Spain

Domenico Rubello, MD
Department of Nuclear Medicine, PET/CT Centre
Santa Maria della Misericordia Hospital
Via Tre Martiri 140
45100, Rovigo, Italy

E-mail addresses:
dfuster@clinic.ub.es (D. Fuster)
rubello.domenico@azisanrovigo.it (D. Rubello)

Diagnosis of Melanoma

Giorgos C. Karakousis, MD, Brian J. Czerniecki, MD*

KEYWORDS

- Melanoma • Staging • Sentinel lymph node
- Biopsy • PET scan

Melanoma is a malignant neoplasm of the skin, originating from the melanocyte. Accounting for less than 5% of all skin cancers, melanoma is associated with approximately 75% of skin cancer–related mortality. Although predominantly found in the skin, melanoma can also arise in mucosal surfaces (anus, vaginal surfaces), ocular (uveal) locations, or meningeal surfaces. Most melanomas are pigmented lesions; however, they may develop from cells that do not contain pigment, so-called amelanotic melanomas. A small percentage of patients present with metastatic melanoma in which after extensive evaluation a primary lesion cannot be identified. One hypothesis to explain these melanomas of unknown primary origin is immune-mediated regression of the primary lesion. Several large retrospective series have reported that these melanomas of unknown primary origin are associated with similar or even improved survival outcomes when compared with their known primary counterparts.[1,2]

Early detection of melanoma with surgical resection remains one of the critical factors determining favorable clinical outcomes for melanoma. This article discusses the epidemiology and diagnosis of melanoma.

EPIDEMIOLOGY

The data from the Surveillance Epidemiology and End Results program estimate the incidence of newly diagnosed melanoma in the United States to be about 68,130 cases for 2010, with 8700 melanoma-related deaths.[3] Although there has been a steady increase in the number of melanoma cases in the past 3 decades (1975–2007), the annual percentage increase has diminished (4.6%–2.6% for the first half of the period compared with the second) and has essentially approached zero in recent years. The estimated lifetime risk of developing melanoma is 1 in 55. The actual incidence of death from melanoma in the United States has remained fairly stable in the past decade (approximately 2.7/100,000) despite an increasing incidence, likely reflecting the increase in the proportion of early melanomas diagnosed.

There is a slight male to female predominance (1.3:1 ratio), and the median ages of diagnosis and melanoma-related death were 60 and 68 years, respectively, from 2003 to 2007. White patients have the highest incidence of melanoma among racial groups, and the prevalence is highest in geographic areas with fair-skinned individuals with significant sun exposure. UV radiation from sun exposure has been associated as the most significant environmental factor.[4,5] The use of tanning salons with resulting exposure to UV-A radiation has also been increasingly linked to the development of skin cancers[6,7] and melanoma in particular.[8] Both the extent of UV radiation exposure and the timing of exposure (ie, early age exposure)[9] seem to influence the development of melanoma. Intermittent sun exposure or a history of sunburns seems to be most highly associated with a risk of melanoma, whereas chronic occupational sun exposure seems to be

Division of Endocrine and Oncologic Surgery, Department of Surgery, University of Pennsylvania School of Medicine, 3400 Spruce Street, 4th Floor, Silverstein, Philadelphia, PA 19104, USA
* Corresponding author. Department of Surgery, University of Pennsylvania School of Medicine, Abramson Cancer Center, 3rd Floor West, 3400 Civic Center Boulevard, Philadelphia, PA 19104.
E-mail address: brian.czerniecki@uphs.upenn.edu

PET Clin 6 (2011) 1–8
doi:10.1016/j.cpet.2011.02.001
1556-8598/11/$ – see front matter © 2011 Published by Elsevier Inc.

inversely correlated.[10] Melanomas tend to occur more frequently on truncal locations in men than on extremities (legs) in women.

There seems to be a familial component in the pathogenesis of at least some melanomas, with approximately 1.3% of patients from studies in Northern Europe to up to 15.8% of patients from studies in Australia reporting a family history of melanoma.[11] Various rare susceptibility genes with high penetrance (CDKN2A, CDK4, ARF) and some with low penetrance (MCR1, the gene considered to underlie red hair and freckles) have been identified, while several others are being investigated.[12–14] Mutations in CDKN2A seem to underlie the development of multiple dysplastic nevi found in the dysplastic nevus syndrome (otherwise known as familial multiple mole melanoma [FAMMM]), which has been associated with an increased risk of melanoma.[15] Patients with FAMMM seem to also harbor a predisposition to the development of pancreas cancer.[16,17] Xeroderma pigmentosum, an autosomal recessive inherited disorder, confers an increased risk for the development of skin cancers, with nearly 1000-fold increased risk for melanomas, likely secondary to an inability for these individuals to properly process oxidative damage to DNA from UV exposure.[18]

CLINICAL EVALUATION AND DIAGNOSIS

The evaluation of any patient presenting with an atypical-appearing pigmented skin lesion should begin with a history taking and physical examination. Particular attention should be given to a history of excessive sun exposure, particularly at a young age, and to any family history of skin cancers, particularly melanoma. The physical examination should not only focus on the lesion itself but also evaluate for any other atypical-appearing skin lesions through a complete skin examination, including the scalp. Attention should be paid during physical examination to the regional nodal basin because a small percentage of melanomas present with synchronous clinically palpable lymphadenopathy. The clinical characteristics of a lesion that should raise concern for the possibility of melanoma can be summarized by the traditionally used "ABCD(E)s" of melanoma:

A. Asymmetry: the lesion does not have a uniform appearance
B. Borders: irregularity in the borders of the lesion
C. Color: heterogeneity in color (variegation)
D. Diameter: lesions thicker than 6 mm
E. Evolution: lesions with changing shapes, size, or color.

In addition, any lesions associated with the onset of new symptoms, particularly pruritus or bleeding, should raise clinical concern for the possibility of a melanoma. More recently, the concept of comparative recognition or the "ugly duckling sign" has been discussed in dermatology.[19,20] This concept refers to the fact that different individuals may have a different nevus pattern, and clinical concern for a particular nevus is based to a large extent on its dissimilarity with other nevi in the same individual and not necessarily on whether it fulfills the ABCD criteria. Essentially, the ugly duckling sign is an attempt to address some of the limitations in the sensitivity and specificity of the ABCD criteria. Melanomas can occur in lesions thinner than 6 mm in size, and conversely, many benign lesions, such as seborrheic keratoses, may have characteristics of the ABCDs of melanoma. Dermatologists rely on the overall characteristics of a nevus, the ugly duck sign, and the subjective change of a lesion as described by a patient.

Dermoscopy has also found an increasing use in dermatology in distinguishing between benign nevi and melanomas.[21] By permitting the visualization of submacroscopic structures not visible to the naked eye, dermoscopy can provide clinicians with additional information in determining whether a particular lesion should be biopsied. The dermoscopic patterns of nevi can be incorporated with other clinical information, such as age, family history, growth dynamics, pregnancy, skin type, and UV exposure, to develop clinical guidelines that can potentially predict with greater accuracy the malignancy of a lesion.[22]

The determination of a melanoma is made by pathologic analysis of the biopsied specimen. Generally speaking, an excisional biopsy is recommended for lesions suspicious for melanoma because this provides for the highest likelihood of obtaining accurate pathologic information that can affect clinical decision making. For large lesions, punch biopsy or incisional biopsies are acceptable methods for obtaining a histologic diagnosis.

HISTOLOGIC SUBTYPES OF MELANOMA AND PATHOLOGIC PROGNOSTIC FACTORS

There are 4 predominant histologic subtypes of melanoma that have been characterized: (1) superficial spreading melanoma, which accounts for approximately 70% of melanomas and has a predominantly radial growth phase; (2) nodular melanoma (up to 30% of cases), which is characterized by a vertical growth phase; (3) lentigo maligna melanoma, which most frequently occurs in chronically sun-exposed areas (particularly face) of elderly individuals; and (4) acral-lentiginous melanoma, which occurs in the palmar, plantar, or subungual locations. Much rarer subtypes include desmoplastic melanoma and amelanotic melanomas (<5% of melanomas). Desmoplastic melanomas frequently present with an increased tumor thickness compared with the other more common melanoma histologic subtypes but have generally been associated with a lower incidence of lymph node metastases and a concomitant improved prognosis.[23] Amelanotic melanomas commonly occur in the subungual locations and are frequently misdiagnosed, leading to delayed recognition and treatment of patients with these lesions.[24] Ulcerative lesions that are nonhealing

in the digital nail beds should therefore raise clinical concern for the possibility of a melanoma despite the lack of pigmentation.[24,25]

Although histologic subtype carries some prognostic utility, with superficial spreading histology typically associated with the most favorable prognosis, other pathologic characteristics of the primary tumor have been identified that seem to confer greater prognostic value. Increased Breslow depth or tumor thickness and presence of ulceration are 2 pathologic factors that have been repeatedly shown to portend a worse prognosis and have been incorporated into the American Joint Committee on Cancer (AJCC) staging system (**Tables 1** and **2**). From the analyses of 30,946 patients with stage I to III melanoma, which

Table 1
The proposed TNM classification scheme for the seventh edition AJCC melanoma staging system

Classification	Thickness (mm)	Ulceration Status/Mitoses
T		
Tis	NA	NA
T1	≤1.00	a: Without ulceration and mitosis <1/mm^2 b: With ulceration or mitoses ≥1/mm^2
T2	1.01–2.00	a: Without ulceration b: With ulceration
T3	2.01–4.00	a: Without ulceration b: With ulceration
T4	>4.00	a: Without ulceration b: With ulceration
N	Number of Metastatic Nodes	Nodal Metastatic Burden
N0	0	NA
N1	1	a: Micrometastasis[a] b: Macrometastasis[b]
N2	2–3	a: Micrometastasis[a] b: Macrometastasis[b] c: In transit metastases/satellites without metastatic nodes
N3	4+ metastatic nodes, matted nodes, or in transit metastases/satellites with metastatic nodes	
M	Site	Serum LDH
M0	No distant metastases	NA
M1a	Distant skin, subcutaneous, or nodal metastases	Normal
M1b	Lung metastases	Normal
M1c	All other visceral metastases Any distant metastasis	Normal Elevated

Abbreviations: LDH, lactate dehydrogenase; NA, not applicable.
[a] Micrometastases are diagnosed after sentinel lymph node biopsy.
[b] Macrometastases are defined as clinically detectable nodal metastases confirmed pathologically.
From Balch CM, Gershenwald JE, Soong SJ, et al. Final version of 2009 AJCC melanoma staging and classification. J Clin Oncol 2009;27(36):6200; with permission.

Table 2
Proposed stage grouping for the seventh edition AJCC melanoma staging system

	Clinical Staging[a]				Pathologic Staging[b]		
	T	N	M		T	N	M
0	Tis	N0	M0	0	Tis	N0	M0
IA	T1a	N0	M0	IA	T1a	N0	M0
IB	T1b	N0	M0	IB	T1b	N0	M0
	T2a	N0	M0		T2a	N0	M0
IIA	T2b	N0	M0	IIA	T2b	N0	M0
	T3a	N0	M0		T3a	N0	M0
IIB	T3b	N0	M0	IIB	T3b	N0	M0
	T4a	N0	M0		T4a	N0	M0
IIC	T4b	N0	M0	IIC	T4b	N0	M0
III	Any T	N>N0	M0	IIIA	T1-4a	N1a	M0
					T1-4a	N2a	M0
				IIIB	T1-4b	N1a	M0
					T1-4b	N2a	M0
					T1-4a	N1b	M0
					T1-4a	N2b	M0
					T1-4a	N2c	M0
				IIIC	T1-4b	N1b	M0
					T1-4b	N2b	M0
					T1-4b	N2c	M0
					Any T	N3	M0
IV	Any T	Any N	M1	IV	Any T	Any N	M1

[a] Clinical staging includes microstaging of the primary melanoma and clinical/radiological evaluation for metastases. By convention, it should be used after complete excision of the primary melanoma with clinical assessment for regional and distant metastases.
[b] Pathologic staging includes microstaging of the primary melanoma and pathologic information about the regional lymph nodes after partial (ie, sentinel node biopsy) or complete lymphadenectomy. Patients with pathologic stage 0 or stage IA are the exception; they do not require pathologic evaluation of their lymph nodes.
From Balch CM, Gershenwald JE, Soong SJ, et al. Final version of 2009 AJCC melanoma staging and classification. J Clin Oncol 2009;27(36):6200; with permission.

helped to formulate the current seventh edition of AJCC staging system, patients with T1 lesions (<1 mm in thickness) showed a 10-year survival rate of 92% as compared with a 10-year survival rate of 50% among patients with T4 lesions (>4 mm in thickness), (P<.001).[26] Patients with T4a (nonulcerated, >4 mm) lesions had a 5-year survival rate of 71% versus a 5-year survival rate of 53% in patients with T4b (ulcerated, >4 mm) lesions. Most recently, mitotic rate, an indicator of the proliferative capacity of the tumor, has also been shown to be an important prognostic factor for melanoma[27–29] and has been incorporated into the current AJCC staging system to further refine the prognosis of patients with thin (T1) melanomas. The 10-year survival rate for patients with nonulcerated T1 lesions with a mitotic rate less than $1/\text{mm}^2$ was 95% as compared with 88% for patients with similar lesions but with a mitotic rate greater than $1/\text{mm}^2$.[26]

Numerous other pathologic factors have been characterized for primary melanomas, but their prognostic significance has been variably reported. The presence of tumor-infiltrating lymphocytes (TIL) has been associated with an improved prognosis,[30–32] particularly, if their presence is brisk, but TIL have not consistently been linked to better survival outcomes.[33] Explanations for this inconsistency include heterogeneity in the patient populations among studies, with studies demonstrating a prognostic role of TIL typically having patients with thicker primary lesions.

Moreover, TIL may be an important predictor of the sentinel lymph node (SLN) status of patients[34,35] but may not be an independent predictor of outcome when SLN status is known.[34] Presence of tumor regression, which is characterized by formation of fibroblastic reaction, has not generally shown to be of prognostic value for melanoma survival[36–39] but has been reported in some series to be associated with a worse prognosis, particularly among thin melanomas.[30,40,41] Neurotropism of the primary tumor, similarly, is not frequently examined in studies and therefore has not been consistently linked to survival outcomes, although a higher incidence of local recurrence has been reported when neurotropism was present in patients with desmoplastic melanomas.[42] Lymphovascular invasion (LVI) has been associated with an increased likelihood of SLN positivity.[43,44] In one recent study, the incidence of LVI in SLN-positive patients with melanoma was 13.7% as compared with 6.3% among SLN-negative patients.[45] In another report examining patients with T2 melanomas (>1 and ≤2 mm in thickness), LVI was found to be an independent predictor of SLN positivity by multivariate analysis, with present LVI in the primary tumor associated with an incidence of 25.5% of SLN positivity as compared with absent LVI associated with an incidence of 11.5%.[38] Clark level, an indicator of the depth of penetration of the melanoma through the various skin layers, has historically been reported as an important prognostic factor for primary melanomas.[46,47] Several studies have suggested that the independent prognostic value of Clark level may be limited, however, when Breslow depth is considered, and this value is perhaps most useful for T1 (≤1 mm) lesions.[48,49] Clark level has been replaced by mitotic rate when this factor is pathologically assessable even for T1 lesions in the most current version of the AJCC staging system.[26]

STAGING OF PATIENTS WITH CLINICALLY EARLY MELANOMA

In the absence of palpable clinical adenopathy, in transit disease, or satellitosis, patients are classified as having clinical stage I or II disease, depending on the thickness of the primary tumor and the presence of ulceration. Radiological studies, such as computed tomography (CT) or positron emission tomography (PET) scans, do not typically play a role in the initial diagnosis of melanoma, which is established by histologic evaluation of the clinically evident lesion.

Further staging workup of patients with clinical stage I or II melanoma depends on the risk categorization of these patients. In patients with T2 or thicker lesions, SLN biopsy is routinely performed to identify micrometastatic disease in the lymph nodes. The prognostic utility of SLN biopsy for intermediate-thickness melanomas (1–4 mm) has been demonstrated by multiple studies. The MSLT-1 (Melanoma Selective Lymphadenectomy Trial 1), a multicenter international trial, randomized patients with 1.2- to 3.5-mm thick melanomas to SLN biopsy (with immediate lymphadenectomy if the SLN biopsy result was positive for metastatic disease) versus nodal observation (with lymphadenectomy for clinically evident disease).[50] The reported incidence of SLN positivity was 16%. The study did not demonstrate an overall survival advantage conferred to the group undergoing SLN biopsy versus the observation group, although a subgroup analysis demonstrated that the survival among patients with nodal metastases was greater in the SLN biopsy group with immediate lymphadenectomy (72.3%) versus the group undergoing delayed nodal dissection on development of clinically evident disease (52.4%) ($P = .004$). Although this subgroup analysis has been met with considerable criticism of not being the primary end point of the randomized study, the results of the study demonstrating prognostic value of the SLN procedure itself have been generally accepted. The 5-year survival rate for patients undergoing SLN biopsy was 90.2% among SLN-negative patients versus 72.3% among SLN-positive patients ($P<.001$).

Although the role of sentinel biopsy in patients with thin (T1) melanomas is more controversial, a growing body of the literature suggests that the incidence of SLN positivity in a subset of patients with lesions smaller than or of 1 mm is sufficiently high so as to justify the selective use of this procedure.[51,52] In one study of 181 patients with T1 lesions undergoing SLN biopsy, the incidence of SLN positivity was 12.3% among patients with T1 lesions that were 0.76 mm or thicker and with mitotic index greater than 0 (ie, mitoses present) compared with the incidence of 5% of SLN positivity in the group overall.[51]

The SLN biopsy procedure is therefore generally considered the single best staging tool for select patients with clinically early-stage disease. Studies investigating the role of PET or PET/CT in patients with primary melanoma have typically demonstrated a low sensitivity for identifying micrometastatic disease when compared with SLN biopsy even for higher-risk lesions, with not an unappreciable number of false-positive findings. In a study by Acland and colleagues[53] of 50 consecutive patients with melanomas thicker than 0.8 mm (mean thickness 2.4 mm), PET scan failed to identify regional nodal metastatic disease in all 14 patients (28%) who were pathologically confirmed to harbor nodal micrometastases on SLN biopsy. Moreover, 7 patients were identified with PET avidity outside of the regional nodal basin. In 3 of these patients, the PET avidity was thought to reflect physiologic uptake in other areas. Of the remainder for whom possible metastatic disease was suspected, 3 patients had positive SLN biopsy results (who would have likely undergone more thorough staging workup before completion lymph node dissection) and 1 patient who had negative SLN biopsy results had further CT imaging that was negative and has remained recurrence free at 1-year follow-up of the study. A more recent retrospective study of 61 patients with melanomas thicker than 1 mm found a similarly low sensitivity of PET-CT (5.9%) for the detection of clinically occult micrometastatic disease.[54] Other retrospective studies have demonstrated a similarly relatively low sensitivity (13%–15.4%) for PET in detecting regional subclinical nodal metastases.[55,56] Prospective studies in patients with clinically early-stage melanoma have also yielded low-sensitivity values (14%–21%) for PET scans in detecting clinically occult regional nodal disease.[57–59] One earlier study[60] demonstrated a relatively high accuracy (88%) for PET in identifying regional nodal disease in patients with cutaneous melanoma thicker than 1.5 mm, but this study did not correlate PET findings with SLN biopsy results, and more than 50% of the patients in this study were undergoing a therapeutic lymph node dissection.

In a study from France by Maubec and colleagues[61] of 25 patient with T4 melanomas (>4 mm in thickness), the sensitivity of PET scan was found to be 0% in detecting microscopic disease metastatic to the regional nodal basin as detected by SLN biopsy. In addition, 3 patients in the study were identified with distant PET-avid sites that did not prove to reflect metastatic disease, and 1 patient underwent a cervical node dissection for PET avidity in the cervical area but was found to have no disease in the nodal basin on final pathologic finding. The findings of this study suggest that even among patients with thick melanomas without clinical evidence of metastatic disease, the role of PET scan in initial staging may be limited.

Although PET scan and PET/CT may not play a large role in the initial diagnosis and staging of patients with clinically early-stage melanoma, these imaging modalities can serve as extremely useful tools for assessing the extent of disease in the follow-up of patients with more advanced melanoma. A recent systematic review[62] of 28 studies with a combined 2905 patients examining the role of PET in melanoma demonstrated a high sensitivity (83%) and specificity (85%) for this modality when patients with more advanced-stage disease were included. The role and utility of PET scan in these advanced settings of melanoma are discussed in greater detail in subsequent articles.

REFERENCES

1. Lee CC, Faries MB, Wanek LA, et al. Improved survival for stage IV melanoma from an unknown primary site. J Clin Oncol 2009;27(21):3489–95.
2. Lee CC, Faries MB, Wanek LA, et al. Improved survival after lymphadenectomy for nodal metastasis from an unknown primary melanoma. J Clin Oncol 2008;26(4):535–41.
3. Surveillance, epidemiology and end results program. Public-Use Data (1975–2007). DCCPS, Surveillance Research Program, Cancer Statistics Branch. Available at: http://www.seer.cancer.gov. Accessed July 19, 2010.
4. National Institutes of Health summary of the Consensus Development Conference on Sunlight, Ultraviolet Radiation, and the Skin. Bethesda, Maryland, May 8–10, 1989. Consensus Development Panel. J Am Acad Dermatol 1991;24(4):608–12.
5. Gallagher RP, Lee TK. Adverse effects of ultraviolet radiation: a brief review. Prog Biophys Mol Biol 2006;92(1):119–31.
6. Karagas MR, Stannard VA, Mott LA, et al. Use of tanning devices and risk of basal cell and squamous cell skin cancers. J Natl Cancer Inst 2002;94(3):224–6.
7. Ibrahim SF, Brown MD. Tanning and cutaneous malignancy. Dermatol Surg 2008;34(4):460–74.
8. Westerdahl J, Ingvar C, Masback A, et al. Risk of cutaneous malignant melanoma in relation to use of sunbeds: further evidence for UV-A carcinogenicity. Br J Cancer 2000;82(9):1593–9.
9. Veierod MB, Adami HO, Lund E, et al. Sun and solarium exposure and melanoma risk: effects of age, pigmentary characteristics, and nevi. Cancer Epidemiol Biomarkers Prev 2010;19(1):111–20.
10. Gandini S, Sera F, Cattaruzza MS, et al. Meta-analysis of risk factors for cutaneous melanoma: II. Sun exposure. Eur J Cancer 2005;41(1):45–60.
11. Olsen CM, Carroll HJ, Whiteman DC. Familial melanoma: a meta-analysis and estimates of attributable fraction. Cancer Epidemiol Biomarkers Prev 2010;19(1):65–73.
12. Hayward NK. Genetics of melanoma predisposition. Oncogene 2003;22(20).3053–62.
13. Harland M, Mistry S, Bishop DT, et al. A deep intronic mutation in CDKN2A is associated with disease in a subset of melanoma pedigrees. Hum Mol Genet 2001;10(23):2679–86.
14. Valverde P, Healy E, Sikkink S, et al. The Asp84Glu variant of the melanocortin 1 receptor (MC1R) is associated with melanoma. Hum Mol Genet 1996;5(10):1663–6.
15. Czajkowski R, Placek W, Drewa G, et al. FAMMM syndrome: pathogenesis and management. Dermatol Surg 2004;30(2 Pt 2):291–6.
16. Lynch HT, Fusaro RM. Pancreatic cancer and the familial atypical multiple mole melanoma (FAMMM) syndrome. Pancreas 1991;6(2):127–31.
17. Lynch HT, Fusaro RM, Lynch JF, et al. Pancreatic cancer and the FAMMM syndrome. Fam Cancer 2008;7(1):103–12.
18. Wang HT, Choi B, Tang MS. Melanocytes are deficient in repair of oxidative DNA damage and UV-induced photoproducts. Proc Natl Acad Sci USA 2010;107(27):12180–5.
19. Grob JJ, Bonerandi JJ. The 'ugly duckling' sign: identification of the common characteristics of nevi in an individual as a basis for melanoma screening. Arch Dermatol 1998;134(1):103–4.
20. Scope A, Dusza SW, Halpern AC, et al. The "ugly duckling" sign: agreement between observers. Arch Dermatol 2008;144(1):58–64.
21. Argenziano G, Ferrara G, Francione S, et al. Dermoscopy—the ultimate tool for melanoma diagnosis. Semin Cutan Med Surg 2009;28(3):142–8.
22. Zalaudek I, Docimo G, Argenziano G. Using dermoscopic criteria and patient-related factors for the management of pigmented melanocytic nevi. Arch Dermatol 2009;145(7):816–26.
23. Lens MB, Newton-Bishop JA, Boon AP. Desmoplastic malignant melanoma: a systematic review. Br J Dermatol 2005;152(4):673–8.
24. Oburu E, Gregori A. Relearning the lesson—amelanotic malignant melanoma: a case report. J Med Case Reports 2008;2:31.

25. Adler MJ, White CR Jr. Amelanotic malignant melanoma. Semin Cutan Med Surg 1997;16(2):122–30.

26. Balch CM, Gershenwald JE, Soong SJ, et al. Final version of 2009 AJCC melanoma staging and classification. J Clin Oncol 2009;27(36):6199–206.

27. Balch CM, Gershenwald JE, Soong SJ, et al. Multivariate analysis of prognostic factors among 2,313 patients with stage III melanoma: comparison of nodal micrometastases versus macrometastases. J Clin Oncol 2010;28(14):2452–9.

28. Azzola MF, Shaw HM, Thompson JF, et al. Tumor mitotic rate is a more powerful prognostic indicator than ulceration in patients with primary cutaneous melanoma: an analysis of 3661 patients from a single center. Cancer 2003;97(6):1488–98.

29. Barnhill RL, Katzen J, Spatz A, et al. The importance of mitotic rate as a prognostic factor for localized cutaneous melanoma. J Cutan Pathol 2005;32(4): 268–73.

30. Clark WH Jr, Elder DE, Guerry D, et al. Model predicting survival in stage I melanoma based on tumor progression. J Natl Cancer Inst 1989;81(24):1893–904.

31. Clemente CG, Mihm MC Jr, Bufalino R, et al. Prognostic value of tumor infiltrating lymphocytes in the vertical growth phase of primary cutaneous melanoma. Cancer 1996;77(7):1303–10.

32. Tuthill RJ, Unger JM, Liu PY, et al. Risk assessment in localized primary cutaneous melanoma: a Southwest Oncology Group study evaluating nine factors and a test of the Clark logistic regression prediction model. Am J Clin Pathol 2002;118(4):504–11.

33. Barnhill RL, Fine JA, Roush GC, et al. Predicting five-year outcome for patients with cutaneous melanoma in a population-based study. Cancer 1996;78(3): 427–32.

34. Taylor RC, Patel A, Panageas KS, et al. Tumor-infiltrating lymphocytes predict sentinel lymph node positivity in patients with cutaneous melanoma. J Clin Oncol 2007;25(7):869–75.

35. Kruper LL, Spitz FR, Czerniecki BJ, et al. Predicting sentinel node status in AJCC stage I/II primary cutaneous melanoma. Cancer 2006;107(10):2436–45.

36. Leiter U, Buettner PG, Eigentler TK, et al. Prognostic factors of thin cutaneous melanoma: an analysis of the central malignant melanoma registry of the German dermatological society. J Clin Oncol 2004; 22(18):3660–7.

37. Brogelli I, Reali UM, Moretti S, et al. The prognostic significance of histologic regression in cutaneous melanoma. Melanoma Res 1992;2(2):87–91.

38. Mays MP, Martin RC, Burton A, et al. Should all patients with melanoma between 1 and 2 mm Breslow thickness undergo sentinel lymph node biopsy? Cancer 2010;116(6):1535–44.

39. Wanebo HJ, Cooper PH, Hagar RW. Thin (less than or equal to 1 mm) melanomas of the extremities are biologically favorable lesions not influenced by regression. Ann Surg 1985;201(4):499–504.

40. Slingluff CL Jr, Vollmer RT, Reintgen DS, et al. Lethal "thin" malignant melanoma. Identifying patients at risk. Ann Surg 1988;208(2):150–61.

41. Paladugu RR, Yonemoto RH. Biologic behavior of thin malignant melanomas with regressive changes. Arch Surg 1983;118(1):41–4.

42. Quinn MJ, Crotty KA, Thompson JF, et al. Desmoplastic and desmoplastic neurotropic melanoma: experience with 280 patients. Cancer 1998;83(6): 1128–35.

43. Sartore L, Papanikolaou GE, Biancari F, et al. Prognostic factors of cutaneous melanoma in relation to metastasis at the sentinel lymph node: a case-controlled study. Int J Surg 2008;6(3):205–9.

44. Niakosari F, Kahn HJ, McCready D, et al. Lymphatic invasion identified by monoclonal antibody D2-40, younger age, and ulceration: predictors of sentinel lymph node involvement in primary cutaneous melanoma. Arch Dermatol 2008;144(4):462–7.

45. Scoggins CR, Martin RC, Ross MI, et al. Factors associated with false-negative sentinel lymph node biopsy in melanoma patients. Ann Surg Oncol 2010;17(3):709–17.

46. Clark WH Jr, From L, Bernardino EA, et al. The histogenesis and biologic behavior of primary human malignant melanomas of the skin. Cancer Res 1969;29(3):705–27.

47. Marghoob AA, Koenig K, Bittencourt FV, et al. Breslow thickness and Clark level in melanoma: support for including level in pathology reports and in American Joint Committee on Cancer Staging. Cancer 2000;88(3):589–95.

48. Buzaid AC, Ross MI, Balch CM, et al. Critical analysis of the current American Joint Committee on Cancer staging system for cutaneous melanoma and proposal of a new staging system. J Clin Oncol 1997;15(3):1039–51.

49. Pontikes LA, Temple WJ, Cassar SL, et al. Influence of level and depth on recurrence rate in thin melanomas. Am J Surg 1993;165(2):225–8.

50. Morton DL, Thompson JF, Cochran AJ, et al. Sentinel-node biopsy or nodal observation in melanoma. N Engl J Med 2006;355(13):1307–17.

51. Kesmodel SB, Karakousis GC, Botbyl JD, et al. Mitotic rate as a predictor of sentinel lymph node positivity in patients with thin melanomas. Ann Surg Oncol 2005;12(6):449–58.

52. Karakousis GC, Gimotty PA, Botbyl JD, et al. Predictors of regional nodal disease in patients with thin melanomas. Ann Surg Oncol 2006;13(4):533–41.

53. Acland KM, Healy C, Calonje E, et al. Comparison of positron emission tomography scanning and sentinel node biopsy in the detection of micrometastases of primary cutaneous malignant melanoma. J Clin Oncol 2001;19(10):2674–8.

54. Klode J, Dissemond J, Grabbe S, et al. Sentinel lymph node excision and PET-CT in the initial stage of malignant melanoma: a retrospective analysis of 61 patients with malignant melanoma in American Joint Committee on Cancer stages I and II. Dermatol Surg 2010;36(4):439–45.

55. Havenga K, Cobben DC, Oyen WJ, et al. Fluorodeox-yglucose-positron emission tomography and sentinel lymph node biopsy in staging primary cutaneous melanoma. Eur J Surg Oncol 2003;29(8):662–4.

56. Fink AM, Holle-Robatsch S, Herzog N, et al. Positron emission tomography is not useful in detecting metastasis in the sentinel lymph node in patients with primary malignant melanoma stage I and II. Melanoma Res 2004;14(2):141–5.

57. Wagner JD, Schauwecker D, Davidson D, et al. Ineffi-cacy of F-18 fluorodeoxy-D-glucose-positron emission tomography scans for initial evaluation in early-stage cutaneous melanoma. Cancer 2005;104(3):570–9.

58. Wagner JD, Schauwecker D, Davidson D, et al. Prospective study of fluorodeoxyglucose-positron emission tomography imaging of lymph node basins in melanoma patients undergoing sentinel node biopsy. J Clin Oncol 1999;17(5):1508–15.

59. Belhocine T, Pierard G, De Labrassinne M, et al. Staging of regional nodes in AJCC stage I and II melanoma: 18FDG PET imaging versus sentinel node detection. Oncologist 2002;7(4):271–8.

60. Macfarlane DJ, Sondak V, Johnson T, et al. Prospec-tive evaluation of 2-[18F]-2-deoxy-D-glucose posi-tron emission tomography in staging of regional lymph nodes in patients with cutaneous malignant melanoma. J Clin Oncol 1998;16(5):1770–6.

61. Maubec E, Lumbroso J, Masson F, et al. F-18 fluorodeoxy-D-glucose positron emission tomog-raphy scan in the initial evaluation of patients with a primary melanoma thicker than 4 mm. Melanoma Res 2007;17(3):147–54.

62. Krug B, Crott R, Lonneux M, et al. Role of PET in the initial staging of cutaneous malignant mela-noma: systematic review. Radiology 2008;249(3): 836–44.

Nuclear Medicine in Early-Stage Melanoma: Sentinel Node Biopsy—FDG-PET/CT

Elif Hindié, MD, PhD[a],*, Farid Sarandi, MD[a],
Soraya Banayan, MD[a], David Groheux, MD[a],
Domenico Rubello, MD[b], Laetitia Vercellino, MD[a],
Marie-Elisabeth Toubert, MD[a], Jean-Luc Moretti, MD, PhD[a],
Céleste Lebbé, MD, PhD[c]

KEYWORDS

- Melanoma • Sentinel node • Lymphoscintigraphy
- In-transit node • FDG • PET/CT • Staging • Follow-up

Estimates for 2010 in the United States are 68,130 new cases and 8700 deaths from skin melanoma.[1]

Nuclear medicine has now gained an important role in the management of patients with melanoma through 2 techniques: sentinel node biopsy (SNB)[2] and [18F]fluorodeoxyglucose (FDG)-positron emission tomography (PET)/computed tomography (CT) imaging.[3]

SNB is a minimally invasive surgical procedure used to determine the presence or absence of occult regional nodal metastases in patients without clinically apparent nodal disease.[4] Best identification is currently achieved by using preoperative lymphoscintigraphy and dual-modality intraoperative detection, using the γ probe and a blue dye.[5–7] Lymphoscintigraphy shows the specific lymphatic drainage patterns. It often identifies more than 1 lymphatic channel draining the skin site toward a regional basin or to different basins.

In patients with early breast cancer, staging with SNB has widely replaced routine axillary dissection,[8] with substantial reduction in overall morbidity from breast cancer surgery. In melanoma, SNB is a substitute to elective lymph node dissection (ELND). ELND of at-risk basins was not a standard, but an optional procedure,[9–12] and was mostly abandoned. SNB offers at least 3 advantages over ELND: reduced morbidity[13]; better prediction offered by lymphoscintigraphy (in previous trials of ELND, the wrong field was dissected in up to 30% of patients)[14]; a histopathologist faced with only 1 or 2 nodes to examine can use serial sections and immunohistochemical staining methods to significantly increase the detection rate for tiny metastases.[15]

Despite these reported benefits, it is still a surgical procedure that is responsible for some morbidity and for generating significant health care costs. Therefore, the routine use of SNB is not indicated for those patient groups at low risk of harboring occult nodal metastases.[16,17]

Procedure guidelines were recently issued by a European Association of Nuclear Medicine/European Organization for Research and Treatment of Cancer (EANM/EORTC) joined committee and

Conflict of interest: none.
[a] Nuclear Medicine, Saint-Louis Hospital, University of Paris VII, 1 Avenue Claude Vellefaux, 75475 Paris Cedex 10, France
[b] Department of Nuclear Medicine, PET Center, Santa Maria della Misericordia Hospital, Viale Tre Martiri 140, 45100 Rovigo, Italy
[c] Department of Dermatology, Saint-Louis Hospital, University of Paris VII, 1 Avenue Claude Vellefaux, 75475 Paris Cedex 10, France
* Corresponding author.
E-mail address: elif.hindie@sls.aphp.fr

PET Clin 6 (2011) 9–25
doi:10.1016/j.cpet.2011.01.001

include a wealth of information and details relating to radiopharmaceuticals, dosimetry, γ probes, and so forth.[18] Therefore, this article is not intended to cover all aspects of SNB in melanoma. It focuses on specific clinical issues that the authors believe should be of interest to the reader, whether clinicians or nuclear medicine specialists. Site-specific imaging adapted to melanoma location is also described, and unsettled issues and new developments are highlighted.

Prognosis of patients with melanoma remains poor in cases of distant metastasis, with only limited benefit from currently available chemotherapy.[19] However, the field is changing fast, with emerging treatments, likely to be approved soon, targeting mutated BRAF or mutated c-kit or based on anti-CTLA4 immunotherapy.[20–22] These promising new agents will probably also be tested in an adjuvant basis for high-risk patients. Improved survival can also be expected after surgical treatment if complete resection of isolated (or oligo) distant metastases can be achieved.[23–26] Melanoma is known to be FDG avid and FDG-PET/CT now has a clearly established role in patients with suspected recurrence for whole-body staging to identify patients who are candidates for surgery.[3,27] However, the role of FDG-PET at initial diagnosis or follow-up of patients with early stages of disease is not well defined.[3]

After a brief comparison of FDG-PET/CT with other cross-sectional techniques for the detection of distant metastases in melanoma, this article examines whether FDG-PET/CT has a potential role in each of the following situations: before SNB; in the follow-up of stage I/II patients with negative SN; before completion lymph node dissection (CLND) in patients with positive SN. At the frontiers of the topic of this section (early

stages), the role of FDG-PET/CT in patients with clinical nodal disease at diagnosis is briefly discussed.

SNB IN MELANOMA
Risk of SN Positivity by T Stage

Patients with apparently localized (clinical N0) melanoma referred for SNB have usually received excision of the primary tumor and are scheduled for wide local excision (WLE). SNB is performed together with WLE.

The melanoma T stage takes into account Breslow tumor thickness and the presence or absence of ulceration of the primary tumor.[17] Breslow tumor thickness categories are: T1, 1 mm or less; T2, 1.01 to 2 mm; T3, 2.01 to 4 mm; T4, greater than 4 mm. The suffix "a" indicates the absence, and "b" the presence, of ulceration. Patients with thin melanoma ($\leq$1 mm) are categorized as T1b if the tumor is ulcerated or if it has a mitotic rate of 1 mitoses/mm^2 or greater.[17] Clark level, which was used for decades, is no longer considered to be a relevant independent factor.

Table 1 shows the probability of SN positivity in patients with apparently localized disease, according to the T stage.[16,28,29]

Prognostic Value of SN Status

A multiinstitutional study examined outcome of 580 patients with melanoma after SNB.[30] The SN was positive in 85 patients (15%). The 3-year disease-free survival was 88.5% for patients with negative SN and 55.8% for patients with positive SN (P<.0001). Multivariate analysis shows that SN status is the most important prognostic factor in patients with early-stage melanoma.[30,31]

Table 1
Incidence of SN metastases according to T stage

T Stage	Breslow Thickness (mm)	Ulceration	SN Positivity Rate (%)[a]	SN Positivity Rate (%)[b]
T1a	$\leq$1	No	3.9	–
T1b	$\leq$1	Yes	12.5	–
T2a	1.01–2	No	10.8	–
T2b	1.01–2	Yes	21.2	–
T3a	2.01–4	No	23.1	–
T3b	2.01–4	Yes	37	–
T4a	>4	No	34.2	37.5
T4b	>4	Yes	55.4	55.8

[a] Data from Refs.[16,28]
[b] Data from Ref.[29]

Because SN positivity increases with tumor thickness and ulceration, the prognostic effect of SN status should be examined in specific subgroups. **Table 2** shows the prognostic value of occult nodal metastases in different T categories. Node status was obtained either with SNB or ELND.[32] Depending on T category, a 9% to 27% (mean 20%) reduction in 5-year survival is observed when occult nodal metastases are present.[32]

Morbidity from SNB

Although the term SNB is widely used, this is a surgical procedure with resection of 1 or multiple lymph nodes with a nonnegligible rate of complications.[13,33] In the Multicenter Selective Lymphadenectomy Trial (MSLT-I), the complication rate after SNB was 10% in the dissected basin (wound separation, seroma/hematoma, infection). There were also 1.5% regional complications (leg edema, thrombophlebitis) and 1% systemic complications (pulmonary, urinary). Morbidity was higher (~40%) in patients requiring CLND.[13]

Morbidity of SNB depends on the regional basin and is higher for the groin. There is no consensus on whether to excise external iliac or obturator SNs identified by lymphoscintigraphy. In positive SN in the groin, the extent of required dissection is also not clearly established.[34,35] SNB in the head-neck region requires specific expertise because of the potential risk to structures such as the accessory and facial nerves. Single-photon emission computed tomography (SPECT)/CT is highly recommended in this region. In some patients with melanoma of the trunk, an SN can be deeply located (eg, retroperitoneal, paravertebral). SPECT/CT is also important for precise location and for documentation.

To Whom Should SNB Be Offered?

In the seventh edition of the American Joint Committee on Cancer (AJCC) *Cancer Staging Manual*, it is strongly encouraged to obtain SNB in all patients with invasive melanoma greater than 1 mm in thickness with no clinically detectable nodal involvement.[17] SNB is also encouraged in a small subset of patients with thin melanomas: those with a lesion 0.76 to 1 mm thick that is either ulcerated or has a mitotic rate $1/mm^2$ or greater (T1b).[17] For this category, the risk of SNB being positive exceeds 10%.[17,36]

Most patients with thin melanomas 1 mm or less do not require SNB and have overall excellent survival after wide excision only.[17]

Patients with thick melanomas (T4: >4 mm) have a high risk of occult distant metastases and were considered by many investigators as not good candidates for SNB. However, several studies have shown that the prognostic information offered by SNB was also relevant in these patients.[29,37] In a series of 227 patients with melanoma greater than 4 mm, SNB identified occult nodal involvement in 47%.[29] SN status was the most important prognostic factor. Five-year overall survival was 80% when the SN was negative and 47% when positive ($P<.0001$).[29]

Knowledge of regional node status is also important to accurately stratify patients in trials of adjuvant treatment. The AJCC recommends that all patients with melanoma with clinically negative nodes and who may be considered for clinical trials

---

Table 2
Five-year survival rates for patients with clinically negative nodal metastases who were pathologically staged after either ELND or SNB

T Stage	Breslow Thickness (mm)	Ulceration	5-Year Survival (%) If N−	5-Year Survival (%) If N+	Difference in 5-Year Survival (%) Between SN− and SN+
T1a	≤1	No	a	a	
T1b	≤1	Yes	90	76	14
T2a	1.01–2	No	94	73	21
T2b	1.01–2	Yes	83	56	27
T3a	2.01–4	No	86	59	27
T3b	2.01–4	Yes	72	49	23
T4a	>4	No	75	61	14
T4b	>4	Yes	53	44	9

[a] SNB is not common practice in patients with T1a tumor.
Data from Balch CM, Buzaid AC, Soong SJ, et al. Final version of the American Joint Committee on Cancer staging system for cutaneous melanoma [review]. J Clin Oncol 2001;19(16):3635–48.

should have pathologic staging with SNB to ensure prognostic homogeneity within assigned groups.[17]

Pathology Staging (Assessment) of Sentinel Nodes

Metastases that are found at SNB are called micrometastases, whereas those identified clinically by palpation, ultrasound (US), or other imaging techniques are designed macrometastases. This definition is different from that used in breast cancer (in which metastases in SN >2 mm are considered macrometastases).[8]

The 3 most widely used pathology protocols for the work up of melanoma sentinel nodes (SNs) are: the protocol from John Wayne Cancer Institute, the EORTC melanoma group protocol, and the protocol of the Melanoma Institute Australia.

Even experienced pathologists may miss 10% or more of tumor-positive SNB specimens when evaluation does not include immunohistochemistry.[38,39] S-100, HMB-45, Melan-A/MART-1, and/or tyrosinase are the most frequently used immunostains.[38] Antibodies to S-100 protein are almost 100% sensitive for melanoma but not very specific. MART-1 and HMB-45 are less sensitive but more specific than S-100.

In the current AJCC classification, the size of the SN metastasis is not taken into account and a positive SN is uniformly referred to as a micrometastasis. There is no lower threshold of tumor burden used to define the presence of regional nodal metastasis.[17] However, measures of tumor burden or disposition in the SN can also place patients in high- and low-risk categories for recurrence and death from melanoma. For this reason, many pathologists may wish to provide information on (for example) diameter of the largest metastasis.[39,40]

Rate of Non-SN Involvement at CLND and its Prognostic Value

The goal of CLND is the eradication of additional disease within the involved basin that is likely to recur, it is to be hoped before systemic dissemination. In most SN+ patients, CLND is negative. CLND detects additional non-SN metastases in approximately 20% of cases.

Several studies have attempted to identify properties of involved SNs and of the primary melanoma that may predict non-SN status. Several factors have emerged as being associated with finding additional involvement, including volume of disease within the SNs,[41] ulceration of the primary, and Breslow thickness. However, it remains unclear which populations may be safely offered observation as an alternative to CLND.

Standard of care remains to perform CLND in patients with melanoma with positive SNB.

Beyond prevention of recurrence, findings at CLND carry important prognostic information.[31,42–45] Many recent studies show that non-SN involvement is an adverse prognostic sign. Ariyan and colleagues[43] found that survival for patients with 2 positive nodes was worse when 1 node was non-SN ($P = .05$). Similarly, examining patients with a total of 2 to 3 positive nodes, Wiener and colleagues[45] found significantly better survival for patients who were non-SN negative than non-SN positive ($P = .0266$).

False-negative Rate: Need for a Uniform Definition

In melanoma, the false-negative (FN) rate is based on the number of patients who have lymph node relapse in a regional basin that was previously explored by SNB and was considered negative. The problem is that some investigators express FN cases as a percentage of the whole population, not as a percentage of node positive cases. For example, in the MSLT-1 study,[46] SNB was positive in 122 patients of the SNB group (n = 764). There were 26 patients who had FN SNB with lymph node recurrence in the same basin. The FN should be read 17.6% (26/148), and not 3.4% (26/764) as reported.[46] When using the correct definition, the FN rates in pivotal series in the literature range between 9% and 21%.[31,39]

FN SNB: Factors Influencing the Rate

Factors associated with higher FN rate of SNB are still unclear. Advancing age is a factor of increased risk,[47,48] probably because of lymphatic dysfunction. Some investigators found that the FN rate increases with increasing Breslow thickness,[47] whereas others found the opposite.[48] FN rates vary with melanoma location: SNB in the groin and axilla is usually associated with high rates of SN identification and low rates of FN results. SNB in the head and neck requires more experience for comparable success, because this region has a dense and complex pattern of communicating lymphatic channels, often with multiple SNs.[7] An optimized imaging protocol, with routine use of SPECT/CT when available, should reduce the rate of FN for the head-neck region.

Technical factors that may lead to an FN procedure are numerous. Some patients may recur in an unexplored basin, or in an atypically located (interval, in-transit) SN, because of inadequate lymphoscintigraphy. SNs can be missed at scintigraphy and/or surgery, typically in cases in which not all potential areas are imaged; in which the node is obscured by another node or the injection site; in which the SN contains too little radioactivity; in which 2 adjacent lymph nodes are believed to be a single one; in which there are false-positive uptake foci caused by skin contamination or lymphatic lakes (focal dilatations of lymphatic collecting vessels). These lakes are usually not visible on delayed images; in contrast, a true SN is still visible on delayed scans.[18]

Lymphatic mapping should be performed before WLE of the primary melanoma, because the latter disrupts lymph drainage pathways and may cause a lack of migration of the tracer or the identification of lymph nodes that are not true SNs.[2]

An FN procedure might also result from massive involvement of the true SN by tumor. Retention of colloidal radiopharmaceuticals in the lymph nodes is based on active phagocytosis. Macrophage function is lost as the amount of metastatic involvement in the node increases. Preoperative US might be important to identify patients with macrometastases. Wound palpation during surgery is required to identify possible large hard nonblue and nonradioactive nodes.

SNB Procedure Optimization: The Role of Nuclear Medicine

Best identification is currently achieved by using preoperative lymphoscintigraphy and dual-modality intraoperative detection, using the γ probe and a blue dye.[5–7,49] Lymphoscintigraphy shows the specific lymphatic drainage patterns. It often identifies more than 1 lymphatic channel draining the skin site toward a regional basin or to different basins. Moreover, on its way to a regional basin, the tracer might be intercepted by an in-transit (interval) node. All nodes draining the skin site directly are considered SNs. Lymphoscintigraphy should combine dynamic and static images. Early dynamic imaging can identify the lymphatic collecting vessels as they drain into the SN. This is important to differentiate true SNs from second echelon nodes that receive the tracer after its passage through the SN. These nodes need not be dissected, thus minimizing the morbidity from the procedure.[6]

When available, SPECT/CT should be used to solve difficulties of interpretation on planar imaging, and is often helpful in melanoma of the head and neck region and of the trunk.

Radiopharmaceuticals used for SNB

Radiopharmaceuticals for SNB are colloids labeled with technetium 99m (Tc 99m). After entering the lymphatic system they are engulfed by macrophages and other histiomonocytic cells of the SN. These phagocytic cells are most abundant in the subcapsular sinus. Continuous transport toward the SNs enables visualization with a γ camera before surgery and intraoperative detection with a γ-ray detection probe for more than 24 h after injection, despite radioactive decay. Smaller particles usually lead to better visualization of lymphatic channels and more rapid SN visualization. However, they might also lead to more diffusion to second tier (second echelon). Large-particle radiocolloids (>200 nm in diameter) are less suitable for melanoma lymphoscintigraphy.[2] The choice of radiopharmaceutical varies among geographic regions and is usually guided by local legislation.[18] Among sulfur preparations, Tc 99m sulfur colloid is used in the United States (usually with filtration through a 0.1-μm or 0.2-μm membrane); Tc 99m antimony trisulfide, with smaller particle size, in Australia; and Tc 99m rhenium sulfide colloid (Nanocis, Cis Bio International, IBA Group, France), with median size of 100 nm, in Europe. Tc 99m human serum albumin nanocolloids (Nanocoll, GE Healthcare, France), with 95% of particles having a diameter less than 80 nm, is often used in Europe. Labeling does not require heating. Individual traceability is needed for these blood-derived products.

Unpredictability of lymphatic drainage from skin and the importance of lymphoscintigraphy

Imaging protocols must be adapted to ensure that all true SNs, including those in unexpected locations, are found in every patient. Patterns of lymphatic drainage from the skin are highly variable from patient to patient, even from the same area of the skin.[2,50] In approximately one-third of patients with melanoma, lymphatic drainage pathways have been shown to be different from those outlined in the early description by Sappey.[14,50] Drainage is particularly unpredictable in melanomas of the trunk located near the midline and in the head and neck region.

Interval in-transit nodes

Although most melanomas exhibit drainage to classic nodal basins (axillary, inguinal, and cervical regions), some patients have drainage to lymph nodes outside these basins. Any node seen between the primary melanoma site and a known node field (interval or in-transit node) receiving direct lymphatic drainage from the melanoma site should be marked as SNs, regardless of its location.[18] The nuclear medicine physician needs to be aware of the unexpected sites in which an SN could be found in a patient and should ensure that all of these regions are imaged.

The definition of interval in-transit nodes is not homogeneous in the literature and this is somewhat confusing.[51–54] However, most investigators[52–54] used the term interval nodes or in-transit nodes to define any hot node that lies outside the usual nodal basins (axilla, inguinal, and conventional cervical groups). For the sake of homogeneity, it might be preferable to use this broader definition.

In most cases, interval SNs coexist with SNs in axillary, inguinal, or cervical basins. The interval node can have a separate channel than the one leading to an SN in the main basin.[51] McMasters and colleagues[52] suggest that hot spots seen on lymphoscintigraphy in a conventional basin concomitantly with an interval site should also be removed. Interval nodes are frequent in patients with melanoma of the trunk as well as in melanoma of the head and neck. In the study by McMasters and colleagues,[52] unusual sites for SNs of head and neck melanomas were hot spots located in the occipital and postauricular/mastoid areas. Melanomas of the scalp often drain to these areas. Other cervical areas (including parotid) were considered conventional. Epitrochlear and popliteal interval nodes occur in a nonnegligible percentage of patients with hand/forearm or foot/leg melanoma, and are often overlooked. Biopsy in the epitrocheal and popliteal region can be technically more difficult. Also, the decision whether the basin should be cleared in case of involvement is unsettled.[52,53]

Nodes in unusual locations can be the only nodes that contain metastatic disease. In the series of Vidal-Sicart and colleagues,[53] SNs outside the main regional basins were detected on lymphoscintigraphy in 59 of 599 patients (9.8%) and were positive in 10 patients (16.9%). Five patients had additional involvement of the regional basin.

Interval nodes that are left unresected can be the site of recurrence. In 1 study before the era of SNB, patients with trunk or head and neck melanomas received lymphoscintigraphy and were then followed to see whether recurrence occurs at the site of predicted lymphatic drainage.[54] Hot spots outside the main regional basins were recorded in 34 of 554 patients. Among patients with visualization of in-transit nodes, 12% had recurrence in the regional basin. An additional 18% had their first recurrence in the in-transit node or in the skin above the in-transit node visualized at scintigraphy.[54]

Lymphoscintigraphy as currently performed at Saint-Louis Hospital

We use either of 2 tracers available in France: Tc 99m rhenium sulfur colloids or Tc 99m nanocolloids. The tracer is injected intradermally at 4 sites around the excisional biopsy site (or residual tumor), at a distance of about 3 to 5 mm from the scar tissue. Skin preparation with topical anesthestic cream is used. The usual activity of radiocolloid is 10 to 20 MBq in a volume of 0.1 mL or less per injection site. Strictly intradermal injection is carefully performed to produce a small visible wheal. The total injected activity is 40 to 80 MBq based on whether surgery is planned the same day or next day. Activity should be sufficient to produce good dynamic and static lymphoscintigraphy with possible additional SPECT/CT.

The goal of lymphoscintigraphy is to accurately identify all SNs, but only true SNs, and to mark the surface projection of them on the patient's skin. Lymphoscintigraphy comprises a dynamic study lasting 10 to 20 minutes, depending on melanoma location, followed by immediate static images. Delayed static images are often obtained about 2 hours after injection. A node that appears in a separate node field only on delayed image is also an SN.

Dynamic phase The vital information obtained during dynamic lymphoscintigraphy in patients with melanoma is the identification of the individual lymphatic collectors reaching the SNs. Visualization of the dynamic phase is made as individual images, summed image, and in cinematic loop visualization mode (dynamic sequential imaging). Cinematic loop allows visualization of the radiopharmaceutical transit within the lymphatic channels, and the location of the first SN.[55] Information provided by early dynamic imaging has the potential to improve the accuracy of SN identification and reduce operative morbidity, by avoiding dissection of non-SN, second echelon nodes.

Static imaging and skin marking Early and late static images are obtained of all potential draining sites for an individual location with an average acquisition time of 5 min/image. Because of the risk of loss of faint nodes (and the radiation exposure to technical staff) we usually do not use a [57]Co flood source to outline the body silhouette. The number and location of the SNs are determined and described after the conventional imaging and, the location of each SN is marked on the skin with indelible ink.

SPECT/CT We complement static imaging with SPECT/CT when the drainage pattern is ambiguous on planar imaging or the location of the SN is deep or difficult to indicate precisely, or when the SNs are suspected to be close to injection sites.[56] SPECT/CT is performed either after the early static images or after the 2-hour conventional images. For the CT part we use low-dose acquisition without contrast enhancement.[57]

We often use SPECT/CT in patients with melanoma of the head-neck region, or the lower trunk. In these patients, SPECT/CT can lead to a modification on the incision (length or site) that would have been planned based on planar images alone in a nonnegligible percentage of patients.[56,58]

SPECT/CT alone cannot replace the vital information obtained during dynamic lymphoscintigraphy in patients with melanoma. The identification of the individual lymphatic collectors reaching the SN on such images is the most accurate method of designating an SN versus a second-tier node.[57]

Report Lymphoscintigraphy images are considered a road map guiding the surgeon.[18] The report includes information on: the number of visualized lymphatic channels during the dynamic phase of lymphoscintigraphy; the number of SNs in each basin where drainage occurred; location of the SNs; identification of SNs in unusual locations, including interval nodes; description of nodes not believed to represent SNs (second-tier nodes, nonnodal, focal accumulations that may cause misinterpretation); information from any additional SPECT/CT imaging.

Suggestions for site-specific protocols
The rates of lymph flow within lymphatic collecting vessels vary in different parts of the body. Uren and colleagues[2] measured the following average lymph flow rate with Tc 99m antimony sulfide colloid (head and neck, 1.5 cm/min; anterior trunk, 2.8 cm/min; posterior trunk, 3.9 cm/min; arm and shoulder, 2 cm/min; forearm and hand, 5.5 cm/min; thigh, 4.2 cm/min; leg and foot, 10.2 cm/min).

No rigid protocol can be given and the duration and camera position depend on melanoma site.

Head and neck melanoma Drainage is slow and the γ camera field of view usually encompasses injection site and all possible draining sites. We perform a 20-minute dynamic image at 1 frame/min. Based on results of dynamic imaging, 5-minute static images follow with optimized detector positioning with sometimes personalized views (eg, vertex, oblique, submental) or optimized patient head positioning (lateral rotation can be useful to position the detector closest to the patient). Delayed imaging allows verification that no other SN has appeared late in a distinct field.

The head and neck is a challenging area. Drainage to multiple SNs is common, and the nodes are often small. The draining SNs often lie very near to the injection site. Also, drainage is often discordant with the clinical prediction. Drainage across the midline occurs in about 15% of patients.[2] Drainage to postauricular nodes often occurs from the skin of the face and anterior scalp. Drainage can also occur from the upper scalp directly down to nodes at the base of the neck or in the supraclavicular region.[2] Lymph drainage can also occur from the base of the neck up to nodes in the upper cervical or occipital area.

We often associate a SPECT/CT acquisition to accurately give the anatomic position of all true SNs. For example, knowing whether the node is located deep or superficial and whether it is within or outside the parotid gland has important implications.[58]

Upper extremity Lymph drainage to the axilla is seen in almost all patients. We perform a 10- to 15-minute dynamic image at 1 frame/min to identify the collectors as they reach SNs in the axilla and follow with 5-minute static images. Skin marking is performed with the arm in surgical position. Delayed imaging should check for an in-transit SN. An epitrochlear node is found in 6% to 8% of patients with upper limb melanoma.[6,53] When considering specifically melanomas of the hand and forearm, Uren and colleagues[2] found an epitrochlear SN in 16% of cases. Other unexpected in-transit nodes are usually located in the medial aspect of the arm (at the middle humeral level). Such brachial node is found in about 4% of patients.[6,53] Drainage to the supraclavicular area can occur in 6% of cases.[6]

Lower extremity All patients have drainage to the groin. We perform a 10- to 15-minute dynamic acquisition at 1 frame/min and follow with 5-minute static images. Imaging can simultaneously combine an anterior view and a lateral view over the groin and upper thigh. (Lateral view is helpful to identify collectors passing to deep iliac or obturator nodes.) Skin marking is performed after early images to best distinguish real SN from a second-tier node. Delayed imaging should check for a popliteal SN. About 5% of patients with lower limb melanoma have a popliteal SN.[6,53] When considering specifically melanomas of the foot and leg, a popliteal node is seen in 8%.[2] Interval nodes, other than popliteal nodes, are rare.[6]

Melanoma of the trunk Drainage is highly unpredictable, especially for lesions proximal to midline.[2,50,53] Drainage can frequently occur to more than 1 of the main regional basins (axillas and groins) (ipsilateral or contralateral) (**Fig. 1**). SNs outside the main basins are also frequent in patients with melanoma of the trunk. Common locations are: the triangular intermuscular space

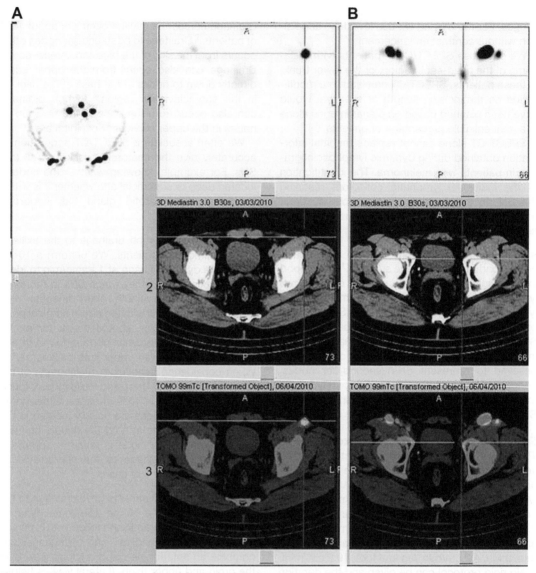

Fig. 1. A 50-year-old patient referred for SNB after diagnosis of a melanoma of the trunk of 1.3 mm Breslow thickness without ulceration, located on the mid-lower back. Four intradermal injections of Tc 99m rhenium sulfide colloid are performed around the scar site. Dynamic as well as static lymphoscintigraphy images (not shown) identify bilateral inguinal drainage. SPECT/CT images are presented. (*A*) Maximal intensity projection image (*left*) shows injection sites and bilateral drainage to inguinal areas. (*B*) (parts **1**, **2**, and **3**): SPECT, CT, and SPECT/CT fusion show the location of 1 of the SNs over the left inguinal region. Secondary drainage to external iliac nodes is also seen.

behind the axilla,[2] the supraclavicular and cervical level V areas, and the right and left costal margins (**Fig. 2**). Direct passage through the posterior body wall to SNs in the paravertebral, paraaortic, or retroperitoneal areas is not rare for melanomas of the posterior loin.[2] Interval nodes can also be found at any point along the course of a lymphatic collecting vessel, and are more common in certain locations, such as the midaxillary line (melanomas of middle to lower trunk), or the upper back and posterior neck base (receiving drainage from melanoma sites high on the back).[2] In the series of Vidal-Sicart and colleagues[53] of 239 patients with trunk melanoma, 36 (15%) had SN in an unexpected location: 28 in the thorax (parascapular, paracostal) and 8 in the abdomen (abdominal wall, paravertebral).

We usually start with a 10-minute dynamic image at 1 frame/minute over the injection site to determine where the lymphatic collectors are and follow

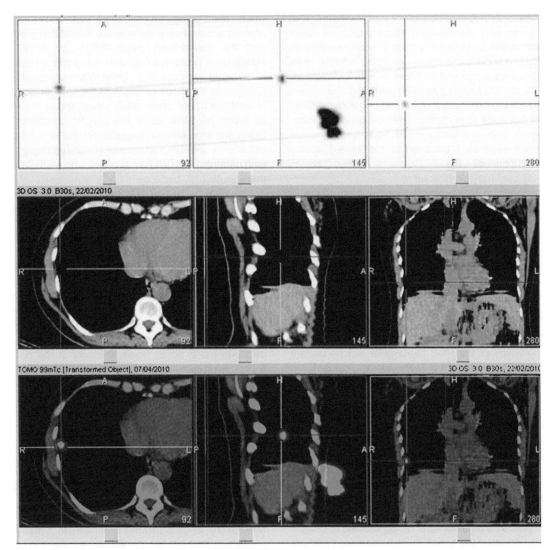

Fig. 2. Lymphoscintigraphy in a 74-year-old woman with melanoma of the right anterior trunk. Dynamic and planar images (not shown) identify atypical drainage over the right lateral chest wall. SPECT, CT, and SPECT/CT fusion images show an intercostal SN. Slight misregistration between SPECT and CT images is due to respiratory motion. Injection sites are visible on the sagittal views.

with 5-minute static images over the identified fields. Delayed imaging is necessary to check for any late-appearing SN. Posterior and lateral views are required to identify SNs in the triangular intermuscular space (located posterior to the axilla, lateral to the scapula), or deep drainage (eg, paraaortic). We perform SPECT/CT for trunk melanoma to clarify planar imaging data (see **Fig. 2**).

Intraoperative Detection of SN

Blue dye is injected intraoperatively just a few minutes before node dissection. Some of the injected dye binds weakly to interstitial proteins, mostly albumin, and this protein binding probably causes the blue coloring of SNs.[18,59] The blue dye travels slowly through the lymph nodes without being trapped. After lymphatic uptake, blue dyes circulate through the venous system to the general circulation. Unwanted effects include protracted blue discoloration, possible interference with transcutaneous oximetry readings during anesthesia (blue discoloration may mimic a true intraoperative hypoxic event), and sometimes allergic reactions such as urticaria and rash, blue hives, and very rarely life-threatening anaphylaxis with pulmonary edema, hypotension, and vascular collapse.[18,59]

The hand-held probe contains the radiation detector, either a crystal or a solid-state device, with surrounding metal shielding and collimation. The analyzer provides indication of γ rays emitted from a given field of view by a visual display of count rate as well as by audible pitch or volume variation. The probe performance is described in terms of its spatial resolution and its count sensitivity.[18]

When a hot node has been removed, the wound site should be checked for remaining activity. Even if 1 hot node was clearly noted on lymphoscintigraphy, in practice this could have been 2 close nodes seen as 1 because of the limited spatial resolution of the γ camera. Deep nodes (>30 mm) may be difficult to localize; image information from lymphoscintigraphy is then critical.[18] Any node appearing firm or suspicious at surgical inspection (large or dark, melanin containing) should also be resected, even if not blue or hot, because it can represent a lymph node that is obstructed or massively invaded by tumor cells.

CONTROVERSIAL ISSUES
Does the SNB Strategy Improve Outcome? Critical Analysis of the MSLT-1 Study

The ability of the SNB strategy to reduce distant failure and improve survival is subject to controversy.[46,60–62] SNB can identify SN-positive patients who can be offered early therapeutic intervention, such as prophylactic CLND and adjuvant systemic treatment. However, there is no firm evidence that either of these approaches results in improved survival.

Melanoma dissemination is considered to occur in either one of 2 patterns.[39] The first hypothesizes that melanomas spread simultaneously through local lymphatics to the regional lymph nodes and at the same time via local blood vessels to distant sites. In this case lymph node metastases are just indicators of metastatic disease.[63] The second suggests an orderly progression from the primary site, through the local lymphatics to the regional lymph nodes, before disseminating further to distant sites. In this case early surgical intervention can be curative.[64] The SNB, with CLND in case of SN positivity, is based on this last premise.

MSLT-1 was designed to test for a survival difference following WLE between patients randomized to SNB and CLND when SN was positive (the biopsy arm) versus observation alone and delayed lymphadenectomy when regional lymph nodes become palpable (the observation arm). The third interim results on 1269 patients with intermediate thickness melanomas (1.2–3.5 mm) were published in 2006.[46] The study reported a disease-free survival benefit for the SNB group (78.3 vs 73.1%; P = .009). This finding was expected because surgical resection of lymph nodes was performed early in the biopsy group and delayed to the clinical evidence in the observation group. Overall, the 5-year melanoma-specific survival rates were similar in the SNB group and the observation group (87.1% vs 86.6%). However, a postrandomization subgroup analysis of patients with positive nodes (comparing SN+ patients in the SNB group with those with nodal recurrence in the observation group) found results in favor of SNB as a therapeutic modality.[46] Subgroup analysis found significantly better survival of patients with SN metastases (72.3%) compared with patients in the WLE-only group who underwent therapeutic LND because of nodal relapses (52.4%) (P = .004).[46] The investigators concluded that "sentinel-node biopsy identifies patients with nodal metastases whose survival can be prolonged by immediate lymphadenectomy."

However, this postrandomization subgroup analysis calls for several comments. FN patients are not included in this subgroup analysis. When including the 26 cases with node metastases and FN SNB, the survival advantage becomes smaller (5-year survival 66.2% vs 54.2%).[46(p1312)] Furthermore, the rates of regional nodal positivity differ between the 2 arms. Node positivity in the SNB group was significantly higher than the rate of nodal relapse in the WLE-only group (19.2% vs 15.6% at 5 years).[46] The excess cases of micrometastases that did not translate into palpable node during the observation period (average follow-up 59.8 months) probably represent a separate entity with less aggressive disease. The 2 subgroups are therefore not comparable.[60] It is important to wait for the fourth interim analysis of MLST-1 for definitive conclusions.

In the absence of clear survival benefit, SNB with CLND should probably remain an optional procedure and not be considered as standard of care but rather an important optional prognostic tool and a means to reduce the rate of regional recurrence. It is also a requirement for adequate stratification before patient entry into clinical trials. The availability of powerful new treatments in melanoma[19–21] should enhance the importance of SNB if these treatments are used in adjuvant settings.

Does SNB Increase the Rate of In-transit Recurrence?

In-transit recurrence is a recurrence that occurs in the skin or subcutaneous tissue between the excision site and the mapped nodal basin. In-transit metastases are believed to develop as a result of a tumor cell embolus becoming entrapped in the dermal lymphatic vessels. They are difficult to treat because they are often multiple and tend to recur.[65,66] In-transit recurrence often heralds distant recurrence. In 1 study, of the 69 patients with in-transit disease as the sole site of first recurrence, 39 developed distant disease.[65]

Some observational studies have indicated that the SNB procedure itself may increase the risk of in-transit metastasis.[67] It was suggested that disturbed lymph flow after early regional node dissection may cause entrapment of tumor cells, leading to in-transit metastases.[67] However, other retrospective studies using multivariate analysis did not confirm these findings.[68,69] Also, in the MSLT randomized trial, the rate of local and/or in-transit recurrence at 5 years did not differ between the biopsy and observation groups (7.7% and 8.4%; $P = .38$).[46]

Although SNB itself does not increase the rate of in-transit recurrence, the fact that patients with positive SN have high rates of in-transit recurrence justifies more intensive follow-up (self- and physician examinations and US screening of the drainage area). In the study by Kretschmer and colleagues,[66] the 5-year probability of developing in-transit metastasis as a first recurrence was 6.3% in patients with negative SN and 24.1% in patients with positive SN. In SN-positive patients with primary tumor thicker than 4 mm, the probability was 44.2%. A similarly high probability (42.2%) was found in SN-positive patients whose primary tumors were located distal to the knee or elbow. The investigators suggest that patients with such high risks may be good candidate for more aggressive adjuvant treatment: radiotherapy to the in-transit area and nodal basins or cytostatic limb perfusion.[66]

The Paradoxic Effect of Age on Melanoma Prognosis and SNB Positivity

The effect of age is complex. Melanoma-related mortality is higher in aged patients. Paradoxically, SN positivity rate is lower.[70] However, the rate of in-transit recurrences increases with increasing age.[65,70] Conway and colleagues[71] performed radioactivity count rate measurements on excised SNs. Counts were lower in older patients, and this was valid for different melanoma locations. Lymphatic dysfunction with increasing age can explain the findings discussed earlier. Slower dynamic and disturbed flow may reduce the probability of melanoma cells reaching the SN and increase the risk of entrapment in lymphatic channel, explaining high in-transit risks.[71]

Can Delayed Visualization of SN Predict SN Negativity?

Some investigators suggested that the time of first appearance of a SN on scintigraphy allows definition of patients with delayed visualization (>30 minutes) who are at low risk of SN involvement and in whom SNB can be avoided.[72] However, other investigators could not confirm absence of risk in patients with delayed visualization.[73] Several factors influence the time of visualization of SN. Melanoma site is 1 factor.[2] For example, melanomas of the head and neck are associated with slower drainage. Increasing age is also associated with slower drainage.[71]

Is SNB Useful in the Evaluation of Melanocytic Lesions of Uncertain Malignant Potential?

The use of SNB as an additional means to help characterize melanocytic lesions of uncertain malignant potential requires further investigation.[18,74]

Is SNB Possible During Pregnancy?

Blue dyes are generally contraindicated during pregnancy. EANM/EORTC guidelines consider that SNB with a radiopharmaceutical can be used in pregnant women with special precautions,[18] although legislation in some countries does not allow its use. When SNB is not permitted, some investigators perform WLE during pregnancy and delay SNB until after delivery.[7]

What Role for US with Fine-needle Aspiration Cytology Before SNB?

If involvement could be predicted preoperatively with US in some patients, SNB can be avoided and these patients would proceed directly to a therapeutic LND. This strategy also has the ability to reduce the FN rate of SNB.

The sensitivity of US has been highly variable and mostly low.[75,76] In a prospective study by Sanki and colleagues,[76] the sensitivity was 24.3% and the positive predictive value 60.3%. When coupling US to fine-needle aspiration cytology (FNAC), the positive predictive value can be close to 100%. However, in the study by van Rijk and colleagues,[75] the sensitivity of US alone was 34% and that of US+FNAC 4.7% only.

The highest sensitivity of US+FNAC was reported by Voit and colleagues.[77] These investigators used targeted US on SNs identified on lymphoscintigraphy in 400 patients with melanoma (median Breslow thickness = 1.8 mm). When US was suspicious for malignancy, at least 3 FNAC readings were obtained, read overnight, and reported before the SN surgery. Considering the 79 patients with SN metastases, US+FNAC achieved a 65% sensitivity, with a positive predictive value of 93%.[77] Sensitivity was 86% for metastases greater than 1 mm. According to these investigators, targeted US of SN identified at lymphoscintigraphy + FNAC might translate into a possible 13% reduction in SN surgical procedures overall (65% of SN-positive patients could be spared SN surgery and go directly to therapeutic LND). Because of the well-known operator-dependent value of US, these results need to be validated in a multicenter prospective study.

Conclusions Regarding SNB

There is currently no firm evidence that SNB with early CLND improves overall survival compared with a strategy of observation with LND at identified nodal recurrence. However, the SN information has an important prognostic value. Results of SNB are also helpful for deciding a risk-adapted follow-up strategy. Also, precise staging with SNB is required before inclusion of patients in trials of adjuvant therapy.

Literature Data on the Role of PET in the Initial Staging and Follow-up of M0 Patients with Melanoma

Melanoma is known to be FDG avid.[3] In patients with advanced melanoma, FDG-PET/CT is more sensitive than anatomic modalities, such as CT or magnetic resonance (MR) imaging, and at least equally specific.[27,78,79] The most added value of FDG-PET/CT is in complementing conventional CT/MR imaging for identifying all metastatic sites of disease before embarking on a metastasectomy of an apparently isolated distant lesion (or oligometastatic disease), or for clarifying the nature of a suspicious lesion identified by other imaging techniques.[3] FDG-PET/CT is also useful in restaging patients who have developed a locoregional recurrence.[80,81] However, the role of FDG-PET at initial staging or follow-up of patients with clinical M0 disease without known recurrence is unsettled. Some of the published results are reviewed here.

Inefficiency of FDG-PET in detecting occult nodal disease compared with SNB
Wagner and colleagues[82] studied 70 patients with clinically localized melanoma. FDG-PET depicted only 3 of 17 positive SNs, corresponding to a sensitivity of 17%. These findings can be explained by the small size of metastatic burden in most SN-positive cases. It was suggested that PET is inefficient at detecting tumor deposits less than 80 mm³.[82] These data have been confirmed by recent studies using hybrid PET/CT.[83] In a study of 52 patients with no palpable nodes, the sensitivity of FDG-PET/CT for predicting SN involvement was 14.3% (only 2 of 14 cases of SN+

were detected). Moreover, the positive predictive value was only 50% (2/4).[83] Thus, FDG-PET/CT is not a substitute for SNB.

Uselessness of PET for initial whole-body staging of patients with localized melanoma
In the retrospective study by Clark and colleagues,[84] 64 patients with T2 to T4 localized melanoma were included. PET examination has revealed no true distant metastasis but 2 false-positive results. Maubec and colleagues[85] performed FDG-PET at initial staging in 25 patients with thick melanoma (T4). FDG-PET was positive at distant sites in 3 patients, but none of these foci represented a true metastasis. Yancovitz and colleagues[86] evaluated retrospectively the usefulness of different presurgical imaging methods (chest radiograph, CT, and PET/CT) in 158 patients with ulcerated melanoma (T1b–T3b). These investigators found only 1 metastatic lesion in contrast to many false-positive results. Thus, preliminary results do not support the use of FDG. However, there are few data on patients with stage IIC (melanoma >4 mm with ulceration), who are known to be at high metastasis risk. Further investigation is needed in this group.

FDG-PET also seems useless before completion lymphadenectomy in patients with positive SN
Horn and colleagues[87] studied 33 patients with melanoma with SN involvement. Positive PET results have been compared with MRI, CT, US, and biopsy when possible and with a median follow-up of 15 months. Nine patients (27%) were positive on PET: 4 cases were true-positive, modifying the stage III to IV. One focus corresponded to a prostate primary lesion and 2 others corresponded to benign false-positive results (thyroid adenoma, benign pulmonary lesion).[87] These results were not confirmed in the study of Constantinidou and colleagues,[88] in which no distant metastasis was found in the initial staging of 30 patients who were sentinel lymph node positive. Horn and colleagues[89] recently updated their series. A total of 80 patients had FDG-PET after a positive SN and within 100 days of the SNB procedure. FDG-PET was suspicious of distant involvement in 13 patients but only 4 were considered true-positive. Four patients with negative FDG-PET developed clinical recurrence within a period of 6 months after SNB and were considered FN. Thus, the sensitivity of FDG at initial staging was 50% and its positive predictive value 31%. These investigators now conclude that, based on the low true-positive yield (4/80; 5%), FDG-PET cannot be recommended as a routine investigation at staging patients with positive SNB.[89]

FDG-PET/CT has low yield at follow-up of unselected patients with positive SN

Data are rare. Meyers and colleagues[90] published retrospective results on 20 patients with positive SN who received FDG-PET/CT follow-up (mostly annual, at 1, 2, and 3 years after diagnosis). In total, 44 FDG-PET/CT scans were performed. These patients also received 28 CT scans of thorax, abdomen, and pelvis and 36 brain MR imaging scans. These imaging studies identified only 1 distant lesion (a brain metastasis detected by MR imaging), with an estimated total cost of $100,360. The investigators conclude that routine imaging added little value in the detection of initial recurrence. Some patients had recurrences that occurred before the initial scan or were detected by symptoms, self-examination, or physician examination.

Although these preliminary data cast doubt on the usefulness of routine follow-up imaging to detect recurrent melanoma in SN-positive patients, the investigators stress that caution is necessary because of the low number of patients.[90]

FDG-PET is useful before lymph node dissection in patients with palpable nodes

Bastiaannet and colleagues[91] performed a head-to-head comparison of FDG-PET to CT in 251 patients with palpable lymph nodes imaged before planned lymph node dissection. FDG-PET correctly upstaged 27% of patients as a result of detection of distant metastases. CT upstaged 24%. The positive predictive value of both examinations was similar, close to 85%. Significantly more metastatic sites were detected by FDG-PET than CT (120 vs 100; $P = .03$). FDG-PET detected more bone/bone marrow lesions. FDG-PET also detected more subcutaneous lesions. For liver, sensitivities of FDG and CT were similar. FDG-PET had lower sensitivity for lung lesions, although not significantly so.[91] In 59% of cases, distant lesions identified by FDG were solitary. Precise knowledge of the extent of disease is important in determining appropriate treatment. Many surgeons pursue surgical excision of metastatic disease if only a few sites of disease are apparent.[23–26] Aukema and colleagues[92] used FDG-PET/CT in 70 patients with palpable lymph nodes referred before lymph node dissection. These investigators used a low dose for the CT component without contrast enhancement. PET/CT results changed the intended management in 26 patients (37%). Distant metastases were identified in 20 patients, lymphatic metastases in another nodal basin in 3 patients, and in-transit lesions in 3 patients.[92] Sensitivity of PET/CT was 87% (26/30); 4 patients developed recurrence within 6 months of a negative examination. The positive predictive value was 97% (26/27). Brain MR imaging was also used and revealed metastases in 5 patients (7%). However, 4 of them had multiple other metastases detected by FDG-PET/CT. Only 1 patient had an isolated brain metastasis, which was surgically removed, and the patient received adjuvant brain radiotherapy. These studies show an important role for FDG-PET/CT before lymph node dissection in palpable node. The investigators do not distinguish patients with palpable node at diagnosis from those with nodal recurrence. Palpable node at diagnosis represented only 15.5% of the series of Bastiaannet and colleagues;[91] this information is not available in the study of Aukema and colleagues.[92]

CONCLUSION ON THE ROLE OF FDG-PET/CT IN EARLY STAGES OF DISEASE

FDG-PET cannot replace SNB because of its low sensitivity. The role of PET examination in the initial staging of melanoma without palpable lymph nodes remains controversial. For some investigators, this imaging technique has no role, whatever the lesion thickness, presence or absence of ulceration, or SN status. It seems that the PET examination has the same low sensitivity in the early detection of distant micrometastasis as lymph node micrometastasis. FDG-PET/CT seems useful in palpable lymph nodes by revealing distant metastasis or lymph node involvement in more regional basins.

There is no consensus on surveillance strategies in melanoma.[90,93] Early identification of patients with isolated metastasis (or oligometastases) to lung, soft tissue, or distant lymphatic site is important to identify those patients with disease who might be amenable to surgical resection. This group of patients may achieve prolonged survival when distant lesions are completely resected.[23] Most initial distant recurrences occur in the first 2 or 3 years.[94,95] A follow-up strategy that includes FDG-PET/CT during this period might be justified when patients have high overall risk of initial distant recurrence. This high-risk group still needs to be defined.

There are only few and mostly retrospective data about FDG-PET and detection of first recurrence in SN+ patients. Preliminary data do not indicate a benefit of routine imaging in unselected patients. However, there are groups of SN+ patients in whom the risk of distant recurrence is substantially high,[94,95] and the role of FDG-PET/CT needs more investigation. Further investigation is also needed in SN-negative stage IIC patients (melanoma >4 mm with ulceration). Prospective studies are necessary. The role of FDG-PET/CT in SN-positive patients should be examined according to AJCC substaging (stages IIIA, IIIB, IIIC), taking into account the total number of involved nodes, and the presence or absence of ulceration in the primary tumor.[17] The effect of additional factors not currently used for substaging (such as size of the SN metastasis, non-SN involvement, mitosis rate in primary tumor, lymphovascular invasion) should also be examined. Identifying high-risk groups who may benefit from FDG-PET/CT in the SNB era is important and would be a logical extension of SNB as a global strategy to improve outcome.

REFERENCES

1. Jemal A, Siegel R, Xu J, et al. Cancer statistics, 2010. CA Cancer J Clin 2010;60(5):277–300.

2. Uren RF, Howman-Giles R, Thompson JF. Patterns of lymphatic drainage from the skin in patients with melanoma [review]. J Nucl Med 2003;44(4):570–82.

3. Sarandi F, Hindié E, Kerob D, et al. Use of fluorine-18-FDG PET-CT scans in initial management and follow-up of patients with cutaneous melanoma. Ann Dermatol Venereol 2008;135(10):691–9 [in French].

4. Morton DL, Wen DR, Wong JH, et al. Technical details of intraoperative lymphatic mapping for early stage melanoma. Arch Surg 1992;127:392–9.

5. Mariani G, Gipponi M, Moresco L, et al. Radio-guided sentinel lymph node biopsy in malignant cutaneous melanoma [review]. J Nucl Med 2002; 43(6):811–27.

6. Thompson JF, Uren RF. Lymphatic mapping in management of patients with primary cutaneous melanoma [review]. Lancet Oncol 2005;6(11): 877–85.

7. Bagaria SP, Faries MB, Morton DL. Sentinel node biopsy in melanoma: technical considerations of the procedure as performed at the John Wayne Cancer Institute [review]. J Surg Oncol 2010; 101(8):669–76.

8. Hindié E, Groheux D, Brenot-Rossi I, et al. The sentinel node procedure in breast cancer: nuclear medicine as the starting point. J Nucl Med 2011;52(3):405–14.

9. Veronesi U, Adamus J, Bandiera DC, et al. Inefficacy of immediate node dissection in stage 1 melanoma of the limbs. N Engl J Med 1977;297(12):627–30.

10. Sim FH, Taylor WF, Ivins JC, et al. A prospective randomized study of the efficacy of routine elective lymphadenectomy in management of malignant melanoma. Preliminary results. Cancer 1978;41(3): 948–56.

11. Balch CM, Soong SJ, Bartolucci AA, et al. Efficacy of an elective regional lymph node dissection of 1 to 4 mm thick melanomas for patients 60 years of age and younger. Ann Surg 1996;224(3):255–63 [discussion: 263–6].

12. Cascinelli N, Morabito A, Santinami M, et al. Immediate or delayed dissection of regional nodes in patients with melanoma of the trunk: a randomised trial. WHO Melanoma Programme. Lancet 1998; 351(9105):793–6.

13. Morton DL, Cochran AJ, Thompson JF, et al. Sentinel node biopsy for early-stage melanoma: accuracy and morbidity in MSLT-I, an international multicenter trial. Ann Surg 2005;242(3):302–11 [discussion: 311–3].

14. Uren RF. Sentinel lymph node biopsy in melanoma [review]. J Nucl Med 2006;47(2):191–5.

15. Cochran AJ. The pathologist's role in sentinel lymph node evaluation [review]. Semin Nucl Med 2000; 30(1):11–7.

16. Ross MI. Early-stage melanoma: staging criteria and prognostic modeling [review]. Clin Cancer Res 2006;12(7 Pt 2):2312s–9s.

17. Balch CM, Gershenwald JE, Soong SJ, et al. Final version of 2009 AJCC melanoma staging and classification. J Clin Oncol 2009;27(36):6199–206.

18. Chakera AH, Hesse B, Burak Z, et al. EANM-EORTC general recommendations for sentinel node diagnostics in melanoma. Eur J Nucl Med Mol Imaging 2009;36(10):1713–42.

19. Eigentler TK, Caroli UM, Radny P, et al. Palliative therapy of disseminated malignant melanoma: a systematic review of 41 randomised clinical trials [review]. Lancet Oncol 2003;4(12):748–59.

20. Flaherty KT, Puzanov I, Kim KB, et al. Inhibition of mutated, activated BRAF in metastatic melanoma. N Engl J Med 2010;363(9):809–19.

21. Puzanov I, Flaherty KT. Targeted molecular therapy in melanoma. Semin Cutan Med Surg 2010;29(3): 196–201.

22. Hodi FS, O'Day SJ, McDermott DF, et al. Improved survival with ipilimumab in patients with metastatic melanoma. N Engl J Med 2010;363(8):711–23 [Erratum in: N Engl J Med 2010 Sep 23;363(13): 1290].

23. Ollila DW. Complete metastasectomy in patients with stage IV metastatic melanoma [review]. Lancet Oncol 2006;7(11):919–24.

24. Petersen RP, Hanish SI, Haney JC, et al. Improved survival with pulmonary metastasectomy: an analysis of 1720 patients with pulmonary metastatic melanoma. J Thorac Cardiovasc Surg 2007;133(1): 104–10.

25. Neuman HB, Patel A, Hanlon C, et al. Stage-IV melanoma and pulmonary metastases: factors predictive of survival. Ann Surg Oncol 2007;14(10):2847–53.

26. Martinez SR, Young SE. A rational surgical approach to the treatment of distant melanoma metastases [review]. Cancer Treat Rev 2008;34(7):614–20.

27. Reinhardt MJ, Joe AY, Jaeger U, et al. Diagnostic performance of whole body dual modality 18F-FDG PET/CT imaging for N- and M-staging of malignant melanoma: experience with 250 consecutive patients. J Clin Oncol 2006;24(7):1178–87.

28. Rousseau DL Jr, Ross MI, Johnson MM, et al. Revised American Joint Committee on Cancer staging criteria accurately predict sentinel lymph node positivity in clinically node-negative melanoma patients. Ann Surg Oncol 2003;10(5):569–74.

29. Gajdos C, Griffith KA, Wong SL, et al. Is there a benefit to sentinel lymph node biopsy in patients with T4 melanoma? Cancer 2009;115(24):5752–60.

30. Gershenwald JE, Thompson W, Mansfield PF, et al. Multi-institutional melanoma lymphatic mapping experience: the prognostic value of sentinel lymph node status in 612 stage I or II melanoma patients. J Clin Oncol 1999;17(3):976–83.

31. Testori A, De Salvo GL, Montesco MC, et al. Clinical considerations on sentinel node biopsy in melanoma from an Italian multicentric study on 1,313 patients (SOLISM-IMI). Ann Surg Oncol 2009;16(7):2018–27.

32. Balch CM, Buzaid AC, Soong SJ, et al. Final version of the American Joint Committee on Cancer staging system for cutaneous melanoma [review]. J Clin Oncol 2001;19(16):3635–48.

33. Wrightson WR, Wong SL, Edwards MJ, et al. Complications associated with sentinel lymph node biopsy for melanoma. Ann Surg Oncol 2003;10(6):676–80.

34. Shen P, Conforti AM, Essner R, et al. Is the node of Cloquet the sentinel node for the iliac/obturator node group? Cancer J 2000;6(2):93–7.

35. van der Ploeg IM, Valdés Olmos RA, Kroon BB, et al. Tumor-positive sentinel node biopsy of the groin in clinically node-negative melanoma patients: superficial or superficial and deep lymph node dissection? Ann Surg Oncol 2008;15(5):1485–91.

36. Kesmodel SB, Karakousis GC, Botbyl JD, et al. Mitotic rate as a predictor of sentinel lymph node positivity in patients with thin melanomas. Ann Surg Oncol 2005;12(6):449–58.

37. Scoggins CR, Bowen AL, Martin RC 2nd, et al. Prognostic information from sentinel lymph node biopsy in patients with thick melanoma. Arch Surg 2010;145(7):622–7.

38. Ohsie SJ, Sarantopoulos GP, Cochran AJ, et al. Immunohistochemical characteristics of melanoma [review]. J Cutan Pathol 2008;35(5):433–44.

39. van Akkooi AC, Voit CA, Verhoef C, et al. New developments in sentinel node staging in melanoma: controversies and alternatives [review]. Curr Opin Oncol 2010;22(3):169–77.

40. van Akkooi AC, Nowecki ZI, Voit C, et al. Sentinel node tumor burden according to the Rotterdam criteria is the most important prognostic factor for survival in melanoma patients: a multicenter study in 388 patients with positive sentinel nodes. Ann Surg 2008;248(6):949–55.

41. Gershenwald JE, Andtbacka RH, Prieto VG, et al. Microscopic tumor burden in sentinel lymph nodes predicts synchronous nonsentinel lymph node involvement in patients with melanoma. J Clin Oncol 2008;26(26):4296–303.

42. Cascinelli N, Bombardieri E, Bufalino R, et al. Sentinel and nonsentinel node status in stage IB and II melanoma patients: two-step prognostic indicators of survival. J Clin Oncol 2006;24(27):4464–71.

43. Ariyan C, Brady MS, Gönen M, et al. Positive nonsentinel node status predicts mortality in patients with cutaneous melanoma. Ann Surg Oncol 2009;16(1):186–90.

44. Ghaferi AA, Wong SL, Johnson TM, et al. Prognostic significance of a positive nonsentinel lymph node in cutaneous melanoma. Ann Surg Oncol 2009;16(11):2978–84.

45. Wiener M, Acland KM, Shaw HM, et al. Sentinel node positive melanoma patients: prediction and prognostic significance of nonsentinel node metastases and development of a survival tree model. Ann Surg Oncol 2010;17(8):1995–2005.

46. Morton DL, Thompson JF, Cochran AJ, et al. MSLT Group. Sentinel-node biopsy or nodal observation in melanoma. N Engl J Med 2006;355(13):1307–17 [Erratum in: N Engl J Med 2006;355(18):1944].

47. Carlson GW, Page AJ, Cohen C, et al. Regional recurrence after negative sentinel lymph node biopsy for melanoma. Ann Surg 2008;248(3):378–86.

48. Scoggins CR, Martin RC, Ross MI, et al. Factors associated with false-negative sentinel lymph node biopsy in melanoma patients. Ann Surg Oncol 2010;17(3):709–17.

49. Albertini JJ, Cruse CW, Rapaport D, et al. Intraoperative radio-lympho-scintigraphy improves sentinel lymph node identification for patients with melanoma. Ann Surg 1996;223(2):217–24.

50. Statius Muller MG, Hennipman FA, van Leeuwen PA, et al. Unpredictability of lymphatic drainage patterns in melanoma patients. Eur J Nucl Med Mol Imaging 2002;29(2):255–61.

51. Uren RF, Howman-Giles R, Thompson JF, et al. Interval nodes: the forgotten sentinel nodes in patients with melanoma. Arch Surg 2000;135(10):1168–72.

52. McMasters KM, Chao C, Wong SL, et al. Interval sentinel lymph nodes in melanoma. Arch Surg 2002;137(5):543–7 [discussion: 547–9].

53. Vidal-Sicart S, Pons F, Fuertes S, et al. Is the identification of in-transit sentinel lymph nodes in malignant melanoma patients really necessary? Eur J Nucl Med Mol Imaging 2004;31(7):945–9.

54. Chakera AH, Hansen LB, Lock-Andersen J, et al. In-transit sentinel nodes must be found: implication from a 10-year follow-up study in melanoma. Melanoma Res 2008;18(5):359–64.

55. Intenzo CM, Truluck CA, Kushen MC, et al. Lymphoscintigraphy in cutaneous melanoma: an updated total body atlas of sentinel node mapping [review]. Radiographics 2009;29(4):1125–35.

56. van der Ploeg IM, Valdés Olmos RA, Kroon BB, et al. The yield of SPECT/CT for anatomical lymphatic mapping in patients with melanoma. Ann Surg Oncol 2009;16(6):1537–42.

57. Uren RF. SPECT/CT Lymphoscintigraphy to locate the sentinel lymph node in patients with melanoma. Ann Surg Oncol 2009;16(6):1459–60.

58. Vermeeren L, Valdés Olmos RA, Klop WM, et al. SPECT/CT for sentinel lymph node mapping in head and neck melanoma. Head Neck 2011;33(1):1–6.

59. Masannat Y, Shenoy H, Speirs V, et al. Properties and characteristics of the dyes injected to assist axillary sentinel node localization in breast surgery. Eur J Surg Oncol 2006;32(4):381–4.

60. Thomas JM. Prognostic false-positivity of the sentinel node in melanoma [review]. Nat Clin Pract Oncol 2008;5(1):18–23.

61. Leiter U, Buettner PG, Bohnenberger K, et al. Sentinel lymph node dissection in primary melanoma reduces subsequent regional lymph node metastasis as well as distant metastasis after nodal involvement. Ann Surg Oncol 2010;17(1):129–37.

62. Pasquali S, Mocellin S, Campana LG, et al. Early (sentinel lymph node biopsy-guided) versus delayed lymphadenectomy in melanoma patients with lymph node metastases: personal experience and literature meta-analysis. Cancer 2010;116(5):1201–9.

63. Meier F, Will S, Ellwanger U, et al. Metastatic pathways and time courses in the orderly progression of cutaneous melanoma. Br J Dermatol 2002;147(1):62–70.

64. Reintgen D, Cruse CW, Wells K, et al. The orderly progression of melanoma nodal metastases. Ann Surg 1994;220(6):759–67.

65. Pawlik TM, Ross MI, Johnson MM, et al. Predictors and natural history of in-transit melanoma after sentinel lymphadenectomy. Ann Surg Oncol 2005;12(8):587–96.

66. Kretschmer L, Beckmann I, Thoms KM, et al. Factors predicting the risk of in-transit recurrence after sentinel lymphonodectomy in patients with cutaneous malignant melanoma. Ann Surg Oncol 2006;13(8):1105–12.

67. Estourgie SH, Nieweg OE, Kroon BB. High incidence of in-transit metastases after sentinel node biopsy in patients with melanoma. Br J Surg 2004;91(10):1370–1.

68. van Poll D, Thompson JF, Colman MH, et al. A sentinel node biopsy does not increase the incidence of in-transit metastasis in patients with primary cutaneous melanoma. Ann Surg Oncol 2005;12(8):597–608.

69. Kang JC, Wanek LA, Essner R, et al. Sentinel lymphadenectomy does not increase the incidence of in-transit metastases in primary melanoma. J Clin Oncol 2005;23(21):4764–70.

70. Kretschmer L, Starz H, Thoms KM, et al. Age as a key factor influencing metastasizing patterns and disease-specific survival after sentinel lymph node biopsy for cutaneous melanoma. Int J Cancer 2010 Nov 9. [Epub ahead of print].

71. Conway WC, Faries MB, Nicholl MB, et al. Age-related lymphatic dysfunction in melanoma patients. Ann Surg Oncol 2009;16(6):1548–52.

72. Cammilleri S, Jacob T, Rojat-Habib MC, et al. High negative predictive value of slow lymphatic drainage on metastatic node spread detection in malignant limb and trunk cutaneous melanoma. Bull Cancer 2004;91(7–8):E225–8.

73. Toubert ME, Just PA, Baillet G, et al. Slow dynamic lymphoscintigraphy is not a reliable predictor of sentinel-node negativity in cutaneous melanoma. Cancer Biother Radiopharm 2008;23(4):443–50.

74. Cochran AJ, Binder S, Morton DL. The role of lymphatic mapping and sentinel node biopsy in the management of atypical and anomalous melanocytic lesions. J Cutan Pathol 2010;37(Suppl 1):54–9.

75. van Rijk MC, Teertstra HJ, Peterse JL, et al. Ultrasonography and fine-needle aspiration cytology in the preoperative evaluation of melanoma patients eligible for sentinel node biopsy. Ann Surg Oncol 2006;13(11):1511–6.

76. Sanki A, Uren RF, Moncrieff M, et al. Targeted high-resolution ultrasound is not an effective substitute for sentinel lymph node biopsy in patients with primary cutaneous melanoma. J Clin Oncol 2009;27(33):5614–9.

77. Voit CA, van Akkooi AC, Schäfer-Hesterberg G, et al. Rotterdam Criteria for sentinel node (SN) tumor burden and the accuracy of ultrasound (US)-guided fine-needle aspiration cytology (FNAC): can US-guided FNAC replace SN staging in patients with melanoma? J Clin Oncol 2009;27(30):4994–5000.

78. Pfannenberg C, Aschoff P, Schanz S, et al. Prospective comparison of 18F-fluorodeoxyglucose positron emission tomography/computed tomography and whole-body magnetic resonance imaging in staging of advanced malignant melanoma. Eur J Cancer 2007;43(3):557–64.

79. Xing Y, Bronstein Y, Ross MI, et al. Contemporary diagnostic imaging modalities for the staging and surveillance of melanoma patients: a meta-analysis. J Natl Cancer Inst 2011;103(2):129–42.

80. Fuster D, Chiang S, Johnson G, et al. Is 18F-FDG PET more accurate than standard diagnostic procedures in the detection of suspected recurrent melanoma? J Nucl Med 2004;45(8):1323–7.

81. Etchebehere EC, Romanato JS, Santos AO, et al. Impact of [F-18] FDG-PET/CT in the restaging and management of patients with malignant melanoma. Nucl Med Commun 2010;31(11):925–30.

82. Wagner JD, Schauwecker D, Davidson D, et al. Prospective study of fluorodeoxyglucose-positron emission tomography imaging of lymph node basins in melanoma patients undergoing sentinel node biopsy. J Clin Oncol 1999;17(5):1508–15.

83. Singh B, Ezziddin S, Palmedo H, et al. Preoperative 18F-FDG-PET/CT imaging and sentinel node biopsy in the detection of regional lymph node metastases in malignant melanoma. Melanoma Res 2008; 18(5):346–52.

84. Clark PB, Soo V, Kraas J, et al. Futility of fluorodeoxyglucose F 18 positron emission tomography in initial evaluation of patients with T2 to T4 melanoma. Arch Surg 2006;141(3):284–8.

85. Maubec E, Lumbroso J, Masson F, et al. F-18 fluorodeoxy-D-glucose positron emission tomography scan in the initial evaluation of patients with a primary melanoma thicker than 4 mm. Melanoma Res 2007;17(3):147–54.

86. Yancovitz M, Finelt N, Warycha MA, et al. Role of radiologic imaging at the time of initial diagnosis of stage T1b-T3b melanoma. Cancer 2007;110(5): 1107–14.

87. Horn J, Lock-Andersen J, Sjøstrand H, et al. Routine use of FDG-PET scans in melanoma patients with positive sentinel node biopsy. Eur J Nucl Med Mol Imaging 2006;33(8):887–92.

88. Constantinidou A, Hofman M, O'Doherty M, et al. Routine positron emission tomography and positron emission tomography/computed tomography in melanoma staging with positive sentinel node biopsy is of limited benefit. Melanoma Res 2008; 18(1):56–60.

89. Horn J, Sjøstrand H, Lock-Andersen J, et al. PET scanning for malignant melanoma and positive sentinel node diagnostics. Ugeskr Laeger 2010; 172(15):1126–30 [in Danish].

90. Meyers MO, Yeh JJ, Frank J, et al. Method of detection of initial recurrence of stage II/III cutaneous melanoma: analysis of the utility of follow-up staging. Ann Surg Oncol 2009;16(4):941–7.

91. Bastiaannet E, Wobbes T, Hoekstra OS, et al. Prospective comparison of [18F]fluorodeoxyglucose positron emission tomography and computed tomography in patients with melanoma with palpable lymph node metastases: diagnostic accuracy and impact on treatment. J Clin Oncol 2009; 27(28):4774–80.

92. Aukema TS, Valdés Olmos RA, Wouters MW, et al. Utility of preoperative 18F-FDG PET/CT and brain MRI in melanoma patients with palpable lymph node metastases. Ann Surg Oncol 2010;17(10): 2773–8.

93. Leiter U, Marghoob AA, Lasithiotakis K, et al. Costs of the detection of metastases and follow-up examinations in cutaneous melanoma. Melanoma Res 2009;19(1):50–7.

94. Balch CM, Gershenwald JE, Soong SJ, et al. Multivariate analysis of prognostic factors among 2,313 patients with stage III melanoma: comparison of nodal micrometastases versus macrometastases. J Clin Oncol 2010;28(14):2452–9.

95. Romano E, Scordo M, Dusza SW, et al. Site and timing of first relapse in stage III melanoma patients: implications for follow-up guidelines. J Clin Oncol 2010;28(18):3042–7.

The Role of PET/CT in Advanced Malignant Melanoma

Imene Zerizer, FRCR[a], Brian Ng Cheng Hin, MBBS[a],
Wing Yan Mok, MBBS[a], Sameer Khan, FRCR[a],
Domenico Rubello, MD[b], Adil AL-Nahhas, FRCP[a,*]

KEYWORDS

- Malignant melanoma • FDG-PET/CT
- Lymph node • Lesion

Malignant melanoma (MM) is the least common but most serious type of all skin cancers, with approximately 10,000 new cases diagnosed each year in the United Kingdom. It has been estimated that the lifetime risk of developing MM is 1 in 91 in men and 1 in 77 in women. Although the incidence is highest in the over 70s, there is a substantial number of cases at younger adult age where MM represents the most common cancer in the 15- to 34-year-old age group.[1]

In the last 30 years, the incidence of MM has increased more than any other common cancer in the United Kingdom. The male rates have increased more than 5 times from around 2.7 in 1978 to 14.6 in 2007, whereas the female rates have more than tripled from 4.5 to 15.4 over the same period.[1]

Therefore, there has been increasing interest in establishing early diagnosis and initiating prompt treatment.

Although regional disease carries an excellent prognosis with an overall 81% and 90% 5-year survival rates in men and women respectively, metastatic disease results in less than 12-months survival.[1,2]

The most common sites of metastases are visceral organs such as the liver, lung, brain, and lymph nodes. Such cases of advanced disease require accurate staging of the metastases to initiate appropriate treatment.

The American Joint Committee on Cancer (AJCC) staging has recently published new guidelines on the staging of cutaneous melanoma and has also made recommendation on imaging techniques used in the staging workup.[3]

Stage I is limited to patients with low-risk primary melanoma (tumor thickness ≤1 mm without ulceration [stage IA], ≥1 mm with ulceration, and ≥1 mm but ≤2 mm [stage IB]), without evidence of regional or distant metastases.[4]

Stage II includes high-risk primary tumors, without evidence of lymphatic disease or distant metastases. Stage IIA includes lesions with thickness greater than or equal to 1 mm but less than or equal to 2 mm with ulceration or greater than or equal to 2 but less than or equal to 4 cm without ulceration. Stage IIB lesions are greater than 2 mm and less than 4 mm thick with epithelial ulceration or greater than 4 mm without ulceration. Stage IIC lesions are greater than 4 mm thick with epithelial ulceration.[4]

Stage III includes lesions with pathologic confirmation of regional lymph node involvement or the presence of transit or satellite metastases. One, 2–3, 4, or more lymph node involvement are classified as having N1, N2, and N3 disease, respectively.

Stage IV is defined by the presence of distant metastases. M1a disease is limited to distant skin, subcutaneous tissues, or lymph nodes;

[a] Department of Nuclear Medicine, Imperial College Healthcare Trust, Hammersmith Hospital, Du Cane Road, London W12 0HS, UK
[b] Department of Nuclear Medicine, PET/CT Centre, Santa Maria della Misericordia Hospital, Viale Tre Martiri 140, 45100 Rovigo, Italy
* Corresponding author.
E-mail address: adil.al-nahhas@imperial.nhs.uk

PET Clin 6 (2011) 27–35
doi:10.1016/j.cpet.2010.12.002

M1b involves lungs; and M1c involves all other visceral sites.[4]

Traditionally, plain radiographs, contrast-enhanced computed tomography (CECT), and MR imaging have been used for staging advanced cases of MM. However, there is increasing evidence in the literature that PET/CT with fludeoxyglucose (FDG) is more accurate in staging of the disease and detecting recurrence.

THE ROLE OF CONVENTIONAL IMAGING TECHNIQUES
Plain Radiography

Plain radiography, mainly chest radiograph, is only used in low-risk patients and has largely been replaced by CECT in the staging of advanced cases of MM.

Ultrasound

The role of ultrasound in staging MM is confined to detection of lymph node and liver metastases. Lymph node involvement is the earliest manifestation of metastatic MM. Several published studies show that ultrasound is superior to clinical palpation and CT in the detection of metastases and in combination with fine-needle aspiration cytology (FNAC) is a highly specific examination.[3,5] Sensitivity for the detection of a positive sentinel node by ultrasound before a surgical procedure ranges between 39% and 79%, and specificity is 100%.[3] In patients with a positive cytology, sentinel node biopsy can be avoided by directly performing therapeutic lymph node dissection.[3]

MM hepatic metastases are typically hypoechoic, with cystic changes indicative of tumor necrosis in 30% of cases.[6] The sensitivity of ultrasound is much improved with the use of sonographic contrast agents that have been shown to demonstrate more lesions and differentiate between benign and malignant processes.[7] Melanoma accounts for more than half of metastases to the gallbladder, and autopsy data show the incidence of gallbladder metastases from melanoma to be 9% to 20%, with a lower frequency for bile duct deposits.[8]

CECT

CECT is the most widely available method for assessment of intrathoracic metastases, which include evaluation for lung lesions and mediastinal and hilar lymphadenopathy.[9,10] CECT is also superior to plain chest radiographs, particularly in detecting bone lesions.[11] It has higher detection rates of purely lytic lesions, which can be missed on a whole-body bone scan.[11] Compared with ultrasound, CT has similar specificity for the detection of liver metastases but has higher sensitivity (85% compared with 57%).[12] Typically, MM liver metastases are of low density with avid enhancement pattern.

MR Imaging

MR imaging of the abdomen has been recommended in the staging of patients with advanced MM, because it can detect additional hepatic metastases compared with CT and ultrasound and differentiate between benign lesions such as haemangiomas and melanoma metastases.[13,14] It has a superior role in delineating the exact location of the lesions as well as vascular and adjacent organ involvement.

MR imaging is the best imaging technique to detect brain metastases, because it can identify very small lesions and give anatomic details to aid surgical management.[15] In the spine, it has the ability to demonstrate spinal cord involvement and leptomeningeal spread, which are notoriously difficult to detect.[15]

Bone metastases can be difficult to detect, and MR imaging may be useful to evaluate bone marrow signal changes by detecting accompanying features such as hemorrhage or soft tissue masses, but its specificity is low.[11]

THE ROLE OF PET/CT IN STAGING MM
Early Stages of the Disease

Several published studies in the literature that included patients with early-stage melanoma showed that whole-body FDG-PET had a low sensitivity (17.3%, range 0%–40%) for detecting sentinel lymph node (SLN) metastases.[4,16,17] A simulation study confirmed that PET-only devices that have a spatial resolution of about 4 to 6 mm have sensitivities of less than 50% for the detection of SLN metastases from MM.[18]

Another study found that the size of SLN influenced the detection rate of metastases by FDG-PET.[19] PET sensitivity was only 23% for lymph nodes of less than 5-mm thickness and increased to 83% and 100% for lymph nodes of 6- to 10-mm and greater than 10-mm thickness, respectively.[19] Another study that compared PET and SLN sampling in patients with MM stages I and II found that 16.7% of patients had a positive biopsy, whereas PET was positive in only 1 patient. The investigators concluded that PET is not an adequate screening test for subclinical and sonographically inconspicuous lymph node metastases in patients with MM stages I and II.[20]

Some investigators argue that MM has an unpredictable behavior, and metastatic disease can occur even in the earliest stages of presentation, particularly in high-risk patients (melanomas of the trunk and upper arms and those with a Breslow thickness of >4 mm, ulceration, and a high mitotic rato).[21,22] Therefore, there is a valid argument for integrating PET/CT in the staging of this subgroup of patients. An example of a case demonstrating the value of FDG-PET/CT in staging is shown in **Fig. 1**.

The new advances in PET/CT remain to be evaluated in detecting/replacing sentinel node localization. Only 1 study in the literature by Falk and colleagues[23] included stage I and II diseases in the assessment of PET/CT in the early stages of the disease, which is described in the section of advanced stages of disease.

Nonetheless, most MM metastases in lymph nodes are only about 1 to 2 mm in size in the early stages of presentation.[24] Therefore, regardless of PET protocols and equipment, metabolic imaging is currently unreliable in the detection of microscopic disease, and SLN localization and biopsy remain the gold standard method of staging local lymph nodes in patients with MM stages I and II.

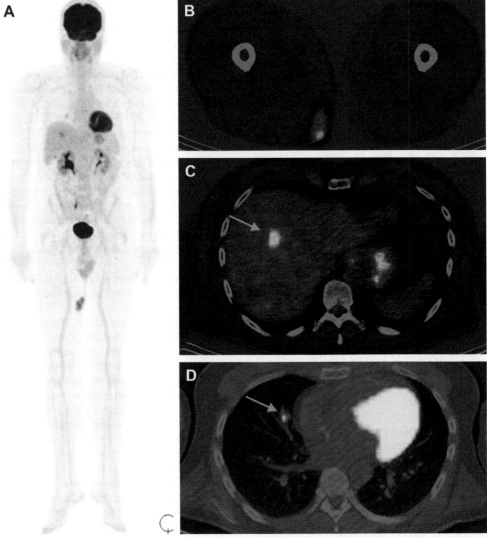

Fig. 1. A 78-year-old woman presenting with a cutaneous lesion in the medial right thigh. Biopsy showed high-grade melanoma. Staging FDG-PET/CT shows a lesion in the right medial thigh, liver, and pulmonary metastases (A) in the maximal intensity projection. PET/CT-fused images show the cutaneous lesion in the right thigh (B), liver metastases (arrow in C), and pulmonary metastases (arrow in D).

Advanced Stages of Disease

FDG-PET has been used in the staging of MM since the late 90s and had proved to be effective in accurately staging patients before surgery.[25–27] A recent meta-analysis of 28 studies involving 2905 patients demonstrated that FDG-PET had an overall sensitivity of 83% (95% confidence interval [CI], 81%–84%) and specificity of 85% (95% CI, 83%–87%) in the initial staging of patients with MM.[28] This figure is higher than the previously quoted figures in the meta-analyses performed in 2000 and 2001,[29,30] which is most probably due to improved sensitivity and technical advances in PET scanning.

In addition, FDG-PET was found to change patient management in 22% patients, and unsuspected metastases were identified in 15% of patients.[31] Another study demonstrated that 26% of patients with stage III disease had a change in their management after PET imaging, with one-third upstaged whereas two-thirds were downstaged.[32]

However, FDG-PET alone has been shown to have limitations in demonstrating visceral metastases particularly in the liver, lungs, and brain.[33,34] The lack of anatomic localization and morphologic appearance can also lead to false-positive and false-negative results.

Nowadays, FDG-PET/CT has largely replaced FDG-PET imaging, offering superior image quality and anatomic information. A large study, which included 250 patients (stage I–IV), was performed to evaluate the accuracy of FDG-PET/CT in N- and M-staging of MM. FDG-PET/CT detected more metastases than PET or CT alone (98.7% vs 88.8% and 69.7%, respectively), and the overall accuracy for N- and M-staging was higher for FDG-PET/CT than PET or CT alone (97.2% vs 92.8% and 78.8%, respectively). In addition, PET/CT was significantly more accurate than PET and CT alone in M staging (98.0% vs 93.2% and 83.5%). For N-staging, PET/CT was significantly more accurate than CT alone (98.4% vs 86.3%). There was no statistical difference between PET/CT and PET alone in N-staging. PET/CT had a sensitivity of 94.9% for N-staging and 98.8% for M-staging. More importantly, this study showed a higher accuracy for PET/CT compared with PET alone in the detection of visceral metastases, particularly in the lungs.[35] Another study of 124 patients with MM that evaluated the role of FDG-PET/CT with dedicated interpretation of the CT component in correlation with histology demonstrated that lesions missed with PET alone were located in the lungs, iliac lymph nodes, subcutis, and psoas muscle. The

sensitivity, specificity, and accuracy of PET/CT for depiction of metastases were 85%, 96%, and 91%, respectively, whereas those for PET/CT with dedicated CT interpretation were superior at 98%, 94%, and 96%.[36]

A prospective blinded study of 64 patients with stage III/IV melanoma compared the role of FDG-PET/CT and whole-body MR imaging in staging disease. The overall accuracy of PET/CT was 86.7% compared with 78.8% for MR imaging. FDG-PET/CT was significantly more accurate in N staging and detecting skin and subcutaneous metastases, whereas MR imaging was more sensitive in detecting liver, bone, and brain metastases. MR imaging was less sensitive but more specific than PET/CT in classifying pulmonary lesions. The investigators concluded that in advanced melanoma, combining FDG-PET/CT with organ-specific MR imaging of the brain, liver, and bone marrow provided a higher accuracy for staging disease.[37]

The earliest PET alone studies have shown that PET was more accurate for demonstrating distant metastasis. A recent meta-analysis of 24 studies (from 2000 to 2006) that were analyzed in 2 groups, 8 for regional staging and 13 for the detection of distant metastases, found that FDG-PET was not useful in the evaluation of regional metastases, as it does not detect microscopic disease, but it was useful in the detection of distant metastases.[38] However, these studies may not reflect the true utility of PET, because they were performed in the pre-PET/CT era, lacking the superior anatomic details and spatial resolution of PET/CT.

More recent studies suggest that FDG-PET/CT was more superior in the detection of regional disease.[23,37]

In addition, a study of 76 patients with MM examined the added benefit of using CECT in the detection of regional metastases.[23] Patients underwent PET/CT with contrast enhancement for staging, which demonstrated that the detection rate for regional metastatic disease was 92% compared with 76% for distant metastases. The trend was significant for specificity: 53 of 53 (100%) versus 36 of 43 (84%; $P = 0.006$) for regional versus distant metastases, respectively. The investigators suggested that the higher accuracy of PET/CT in the detection of regional metastases is due to the improved anatomic resolution achieved with PET/CT when combined with diagnostic CECT. They, therefore, concluded that although PET may be more superior in the detection of distant metastases, PET/CT was more suitable for small anatomic parts such as lymph nodes.[23]

New data indicate that PET/CT may be the most accurate test for the diagnosis of bone metastases.[3]

The current protocol for performing PET/CT at most institutions consists of scanning the whole body from vertex to feet. This is in accordance with protocols in several published studies.[23,36] However, a study that evaluated the value of including the brain and the extremities during PET/CT scanning of patients with no known or suspected primary or metastatic MM found no additional benefit.[39] The investigators suggested that skull base to upper thigh scan protocol suffices for this group of patients. Although this may be a valid protocol in a small/busy department, the recent advances in PET/CT acquisition allows faster scans to be performed, and inclusion of extremities and brain at the institution increases the scanning time only by 15 minutes.

Influence of PET/CT on Management

Falk and colleagues[23] found in their cohort that 27.6% of the patients who underwent a PET/CT had a change in management. Change of treatment occurred most frequently in patients presenting for staging. The impact of FDG-PET on surgical management of patients with melanoma was investigated in a retrospective review of 257 patients with stage III and IV disease. Twenty two percent of the patients were upstaged as a result of PET findings, and in 17.1% the treatment was changed from surgery to systemic therapy.[40]

Prior studies and a meta-analysis of 8 studies suggested that the overall change in management was 33% (range 15%–64%).[28] Reinhardt and colleagues[35] found that PET/CT altered management in 48.4% of their patients.

THE ROLE OF PET/CT IN RECURRENCE AND FOLLOW-UP

A few studies in the literature have evaluated the role of FDG-PET/CT in detecting recurrence. The role of PET and conventional imaging (plain radiography, CT, ultrasound, and brain MR imaging) were compared in a study of 156 patients with suspected melanoma recurrence.[41] The sensitivity and specificity of PET for diagnosing recurrence were 74% and 86%, respectively. These were significantly higher than those obtained with conventional imaging, which had a sensitivity of only 58% and a specificity of 45%. PET was more accurate than CT in detecting recurrence in the skin, lymph nodes, abdomen, liver, and bone metastases. The accuracy of PET for lung parenchymal lesions was similar to that of CT. Although

CT was more sensitive than PET (93% vs 57%) in cases with pulmonary metastases, PET was more specific (92% vs 70%).[41]

Another retrospective study of 106 patients with MM restaging for suspected recurrence found that FDG-PET/CT had a sensitivity of 89.3% and a specificity of 88% for detection of recurrent melanoma.[42] The investigators suggested that PET/CT should be an integral part in the evaluation of patients with high-risk melanoma recurrence.[42]

It has also been suggested in the literature that standardized uptake value (SUV) or level of metabolic activity at initial diagnosis is a predictor of outcome in the follow-up of patients with MM. A study of 38 patients with MM who presented with lymph node metastases demonstrated that the level of FDG uptake using SUVmean predicted risk for recurrence. Disease-free survival of patients with melanoma was prolonged in those with a low SUVmean value in their lymph node metastasis, as compared with those with a high SUVmean. However, this difference was not significant for overall survival. In their multivariate analysis, the investigators found that a high SUVmean was an independent prognostic factor for disease-free survival.[40]

A few studies have investigated the use of PET for routine surveillance or therapeutic monitoring. A recent study of 25 patients with stage IV disease evaluated the role of PET/CT, CT, MR imaging, and S-100B tumor marker.[43] FDG-PET/CT and S-100B after 3 cycles of chemotherapy was compared with baseline PET/CT and baseline S-100B. Patients also had CT and MR imaging of the brain. There was agreement between FDG-PET/CT and CT response assessment. Longer overall survival (OS) was found in PET/CT responders compared with PET/CT nonresponders (80% 1-year OS vs 40%). There was also significant longer progression free survival (PFS) in patients who were found have PET/CT negative result. Chemotherapy response assessment with S-100B failed to show correlation with OS or PFS. There was a higher detection rate of brain metastases with MR imaging compared with PET/CT.[43]

A study by the same investigators that evaluated the role of FDG-PET/CT in patients with MM followed up with S-100B in 165 patients found that PET/CT identified correctly the presence of recurrent disease in all patients except one and excluded the presence of metastases in all patients.[36] Therefore, the sensitivity for PET/CT to detect recurrence in the presence of elevated S-100B was 96% and specificity 100%. These figures were higher for distant metastases compared with regional lymph node recurrence. They suggested that the latter finding may be due to the small volume of the local recurrence resulting in underestimation of SUV and partial volume effect.[36] The authors also found that PET/CT did not miss any cases of brain metastases. However, they recommend a brain MR imaging in the presence of elevated serum S-100B and a negative PET/CT result. Examples of cases demonstrating the value of FDG-PET/CT in recurrent disease are shown in **Figs. 2** and **3**.

Advances in PET/CT in MM

There are few studies in the literature that investigated the role of different PET/CT tracers or novel PET/CT techniques in imaging MM. In one study, the feasibility of 3'-^{18}F-fluoro-3'-deoxy-L-thymidine PET (FLT-PET) for staging patients with clinical stage III melanoma was investigated. Only 10 patients with metastatic (clinical stage III) MM were included. A whole-body FLT-PET was performed, and the results correlated with histopathological findings of dissected lymph node. All locoregional metastases were correctly visualized by FLT-PET. However, there were 2 false-positive lesions giving a sensitivity of 88%. The detection limit for lymph node metastases in this study was 6 mm. Two patients were upstaged by FLT-PET, which was confirmed by CT. In addition, FLT-PET detected unexpected sites of metastases in 3 patients that were initially missed by clinical staging. The investigators concluded that FLT-PET was a promising agent for staging patients with stage III MM, but further extensive research was required.

The role of dual-time-point imaging with FDG-PET/CT has not been evaluated yet in MM. There is evidence in the literature that this technique is more sensitive for the detection of liver metastases by improving tumor-to-background ratio, resulting in an increase in hypermetabolic lesion diameter.[44] This seems to be a promising technique that could be used in detecting visceral metastases in MM, which some investigators have suggested are missed by FDG-PET/CT.

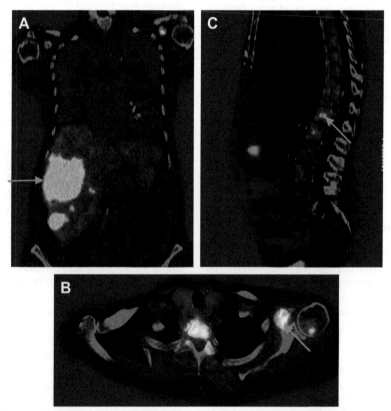

Fig. 2. A 75-year-old woman was diagnosed with melanoma 20 years ago and treated with excision. She presented recently with liver and bony lesions suspicious for recurrence. A whole-body FDG-PET/CT was performed showing extensive liver metastases in the coronal sections (*arrow in A*) and multiple bony lesions in the transverse (*arrow in B*) and sagittal (*arrow in C*) sections.

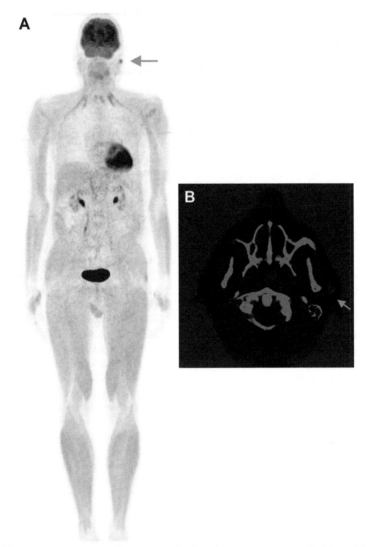

Fig. 3. A 61-year-old man with a previous diagnosis of forehead melanoma, treated with excision, presented with a lump in front of his left ear. FDG-PET/CT demonstrates an active preauricular lymph node in the maximum intensity projection image (*A*) and fused transverse sections (*arrow in B*), which was confirmed to be a recurrence on biopsy.

SUMMARY

In conclusion, FDG-PET/CT demonstrates a high sensitivity and specificity for detecting both locoregional and distant metastases in patients presenting with AJCC stages III and IV disease. PET/CT seemed to be more precise than PET alone. The addition of CT has allowed the detection of pulmonary metastases and improved anatomic localization of other sites of metastases. The use of CECT may be even more useful particularly in the detection of liver and brain metastases. However, currently this may not be applicable to all PET/CT units, and brain MR imaging/contrast CT should still be performed when brain or liver metastases are suspected. PET/CT also plays an important role in the detection of recurrence particularly in high-risk group patients, and this should be the modality of choice in investigating patients for suspected recurrence. The role of PET/CT in response assessment and follow-up still has to be defined, and cost-effectiveness analysis is required to strength its role.

In AJCC stages I and II, some patients may also benefit from undergoing FDG-PET/CT, but there is no strong evidence in the literature to support its effectiveness. Therefore, the selection of patients with early stages of the disease to undergo PET/CT scanning should be performed on a patient-to-patient basis. Larger prospective studies are warranted to assess changes in patient management as a result of PET/CT in this subgroup.

Overall, PET/CT is more accurate than CT or MR imaging alone in the diagnosis of metastasis, but further studies are required to evaluate its role in response assessment, follow-up, and improved patient outcome.

REFERENCES

1. Cancer research. 2010. Available at: http://info.cancerresearchuk.org/cancerstats/types/skin/incidence/index.htm. Accessed December 13, 2010.

2. Wagner JD, Davidson D, Coleman JJ III, et al. Lymph node tumor volumes in patients undergoing sentinel lymph node biopsy for cutaneous melanoma. Ann Surg Oncol 1999;6(4):398–404.

3. Mohr P, Eggermont AM, Hauschild A, et al. Staging of cutaneous melanoma. Ann Oncol 2009;20(Suppl 6):vi14–21.

4. Hafner J, Schmid MH, Kempf W, et al. Baseline staging in cutaneous malignant melanoma. Br J Dermatol 2004;150(4):677–86.

5. Rossi CR, Mocellin S, Scagnet B, et al. The role of preoperative ultrasound scan in detecting lymph node metastasis before sentinel node biopsy in melanoma patients. J Surg Oncol 2003;83(2):80–4.

6. Paling MR, Shawker TH, Love IL. The sonographic appearance of metastatic malignant melanoma. J Ultrasound Med 1982;1(2):75–8.

7. Dietrich CF. Characterisation of focal liver lesions with contrast enhanced ultrasonography. Eur J Radiol 2004;51(Suppl):S9–17.

8. Backman H. Metastases of malignant melanoma in the gastrointestinal tract. Geriatrics 1969;24(8):112–20.

9. Kostrubiak I, Whitley NO, Aisner J, et al. The use of computed body tomography in malignant melanoma. JAMA 1988;259(19):2896–7.

10. Heaston DK, Putman CE, Rodan BA, et al. Solitary pulmonary metastases in high-risk melanoma patients: a prospective comparison of conventional and computed tomography. AJR Am J Roentgenol 1983;141(1):169–74.

11. drup-Link HE, Franzius C, Link TM, et al. Whole-body MR imaging for detection of bone metastases in children and young adults: comparison with skeletal scintigraphy and FDG PET. AJR Am J Roentgenol 2001;177(1):229–36.

12. Kaufmann PM, Crone-Munzebrock W. [Tumor follow-up using sonography and computed tomography in the abdominal region of patients with malignant melanoma]. Aktuelle Radiol 1992;2(2):81–5 [in German].

13. Paley MR, Ros PR. Hepatic metastases. Radiol Clin North Am 1998;36(2):349–63.

14. Ghanem N, Altehoefer C, Hogerle S, et al. Detectability of liver metastases in malignant melanoma: prospective comparison of magnetic resonance imaging and positron emission tomography. Eur J Radiol 2005;54(2):264–70.

15. Aukema TS, Valdes Olmos RA, Wouters MW, et al. Utility of Preoperative 18F-FDG PET/CT and brain MRI in melanoma patients with palpable lymph node metastases. Ann Surg Oncol 2010;17(10):2773–8.

16. Belhocine T, Pierard G, De Labrassinne M, et al. Staging of regional nodes in AJCC stage I and II melanoma: 18FDG PET imaging versus sentinel node detection. Oncologist 2002;7(4):271–8.

17. Havenga K, Cobben DC, Oyen WJ, et al. Fluorodeoxyglucose-positron emission tomography and sentinel lymph node biopsy in staging primary cutaneous melanoma. Eur J Surg Oncol 2003;29(8):662–4.

18. Mijnhout GS, Hoekstra OS, van LA, et al. How morphometric analysis of metastatic load predicts the (un)usefulness of PET scanning: the case of lymph node staging in melanoma. J Clin Pathol 2003;56(4):283–6.

19. Crippa F, Leutner M, Belli F, et al. Which kinds of lymph node metastases can FDG PET detect? A clinical study in melanoma. J Nucl Med 2000;41(9):1491–4.

20. Fink AM, Holle-Robatsch S, Herzog N, et al. Positron emission tomography is not useful in detecting metastasis in the sentinel lymph node in patients with primary malignant melanoma stage I and II. Melanoma Res 2004;14(2):141–5.

21. Vereecken P, Laporte M, Petein M, et al. Evaluation of extensive initial staging procedure in intermediate/high-risk melanoma patients. J Eur Acad Dermatol Venereol 2005;19(1):66–73.

22. Belhocine TZ, Scott AM, Even-Sapir E, et al. Role of nuclear medicine in the management of cutaneous malignant melanoma. J Nucl Med 2006;47(6):957–67.

23. Falk MS, Truitt AK, Coakley FV, et al. Interpretation, accuracy and management implications of FDG PET/CT in cutaneous malignant melanoma. Nucl Med Commun 2007;28(4):273–80.

24. Wagner JD, Schauwecker DS, Davidson D, et al. FDG-PET sensitivity for melanoma lymph node metastases is dependent on tumor volume. J Surg Oncol 2001;77(4):237–42.

25. Gritters LS, Francis IR, Zasadny KR, et al. Initial assessment of positron emission tomography using 2-fluorine-18-fluoro-2-deoxy-D-glucose in the imaging of malignant melanoma. J Nucl Med 1993;34(9):1420–7.

26. Holder WD Jr, White RL Jr, Zuger JH, et al. Effectiveness of positron emission tomography for the detection of melanoma metastases. Ann Surg 1998;227(5):764–9.

27. Rinne D, Baum RP, Hor G, et al. Primary staging and follow-up of high risk melanoma patients with whole-body 18F-fluorodeoxyglucose positron emission

tomography: results of a prospective study of 100 patients. Cancer 1998;82(9):1664–71.

28. Krug B, Crott R, Lonneux M, et al. Role of PET in the initial staging of cutaneous malignant melanoma: systematic review. Radiology 2008;249(3):836–44.

29. Schwimmer J, Essner R, Patel A, et al. A review of the literature for whole-body FDG PET in the management of patients with melanoma. Q J Nucl Med 2000;44(2):153–67.

30. Mijnhout GS, Hoekstra OS, van Tulder MW, et al. Systematic review of the diagnostic accuracy of (18)F-fluorodeoxyglucose positron emission tomography in melanoma patients. Cancer 2001;91(8): 1530–42.

31. Tyler DS, Onaitis M, Kherani A, et al. Positron emission tomography scanning in malignant melanoma. Cancer 2000;89(5):1019–25.

32. Stas M, Stroobants S, Dupont P, et al. 18-FDG PET scan in the staging of recurrent melanoma: additional value and therapeutic impact. Melanoma Res 2002;12(5):479–90.

33. Swetter SM, Carroll LA, Johnson DL, et al. Positron emission tomography is superior to computed tomography for metastatic detection in melanoma patients. Ann Surg Oncol 2002;9(7):646–53.

34. Gulec SA, Faries MB, Lee CC, et al. The role of fluorine-18 deoxyglucose positron emission tomography in the management of patients with metastatic melanoma: impact on surgical decision making. Clin Nucl Med 2003;28(12):961–5.

35. Reinhardt MJ, Joe AY, Jaeger U, et al. Diagnostic performance of whole body dual modality 18F-FDG PET/CT imaging for N- and M-staging of malignant melanoma: experience with 250 consecutive patients. J Clin Oncol 2006;24(7):1178–87.

36. Strobel K, Dummer R, Husarik DB, et al. High-risk melanoma: accuracy of FDG PET/CT with added

CT morphologic information for detection of metastases. Radiology 2007;244(2):566–74.

37. Pfannenberg C, Aschoff P, Schanz S, et al. Prospective comparison of 18F-fluorodeoxyglucose positron emission tomography/computed tomography and whole-body magnetic resonance imaging in staging of advanced malignant melanoma. Eur J Cancer 2007;43(3):557–64.

38. Jimenez-Requena F, gado-Bolton RC, Fernandez-Perez C, et al. Meta-analysis of the performance of (18)F-FDG PET in cutaneous melanoma. Eur J Nucl Med Mol Imaging 2010;37(2):284–300.

39. Niederkohr RD, Rosenberg J, Shabo G, et al. Clinical value of including the head and lower extremities in 18F-FDG PET/CT imaging for patients with malignant melanoma. Nucl Med Commun 2007; 28(9):688–95.

40. Bastiaannet E, Oyen WJ, Meijer S, et al. Impact of [18F]fluorodeoxyglucose positron emission tomography on surgical management of melanoma patients. Br J Surg 2006;93(2):243–9.

41. Fuster D, Chiang S, Johnson G, et al. Is 18F-FDG PET more accurate than standard diagnostic procedures in the detection of suspected recurrent melanoma? J Nucl Med 2004;45(8):1323–7.

42. Iagaru A, Quon A, Johnson D, et al. 2-Deoxy-2-[F-18]fluoro-D-glucose positron emission tomography/computed tomography in the management of melanoma. Mol Imaging Biol 2007;9(1):50–7.

43. Strobel K, Dummer R, Steinert HC, et al. Chemotherapy response assessment in stage IV melanoma patients-comparison of 18F-FDG-PET/CT, CT, brain MRI, and tumormarker S-100B. Eur J Nucl Med Mol Imaging 2008;35(10):1786–95.

44. Dirisamer A, Halpern BS, Schima W, et al. Dual-time-point FDG-PET/CT for the detection of hepatic metastases. Mol Imaging Biol 2008;10(6):335–40.

Advanced Stages of Melanoma: Role of Structural Imaging

Justin E. Mackey, MD[a], Drew A. Torigian, MD, MA[b],*

KEYWORDS

• Melanoma • Structural imaging • CT • MRI

In recent years, the incidence of malignant melanoma has increased at a rate greater than any other cancer occurring in humans. In the United States, the incidence of invasive melanoma continues to increase 4% to 6% annually despite efforts to improve primary prevention. Similar increases are being seen worldwide. It is estimated that 68,720 Americans were diagnosed as having melanoma in 2009, and that the current lifetime risk for developing invasive melanoma is 1 in 58. When the estimated 53,120 cases of in situ melanoma are added, the lifetime risk for a diagnosis of melanoma is 1 in 30. It was also estimated that 8650 Americans died of melanoma in 2009.[1,2]

The prognosis of patients with melanoma is strongly related to the stage at detection.[3] The 5-year survival for patients with stage III melanoma according to the American Joint Committee on Cancer classification is as low as 40%, and the 1-year survival for patients with stage IV melanoma is as low as 33%, respectively.[4] A complete nodal dissection in stage III disease and resection of metastases in cases of limited stage IV disease are probably the most effective methods in prolonging survival.[5] Therefore, it is essential to be able to reliably detect the presence of advanced disease to guide treatment strategies and to predict patient prognosis.

USEFULNESS OF STRUCTURAL IMAGING

Complete evaluation of tumor spread requires the use of various imaging modalities, including computed tomography (CT), magnetic resonance (MR) imaging, ultrasonography (US), radiography, scintigraphy, and positron emission tomography (PET). Each modality has its advantages and disadvantages, and it is important to understand these to maximize their usefulness in patient management. This article focuses primarily on structural imaging with an emphasis on CT and MR imaging, with some mention of US, because these are the structural imaging modalities most often used today.

CT and MR imaging both have advantages of high spatial resolution, multiplanar tomographic or volumetric image display, relatively good soft-tissue contrast between normal structures and disease processes, relatively short examination times (typically <5–10 minutes for CT and <20–30 minutes for MR imaging), and the capability for whole-body imaging (related to multidetector row and parallel imaging technologies, respectively). CT has higher spatial resolution than MR imaging, has superior sensitivity for detection of calcification, ossification, or gas compared with MR imaging, and can be used when there are contraindications to MR imaging, such as the presence of a transvenous pacemaker, intracranial ferromagnetic aneurysm clips, or orbital metallic foreign bodies. MR imaging does not use ionizing radiation, has superior contrast resolution compared with CT, can be used when there are contraindications to performance of an iodinated contrast-enhanced CT (such as an iodinated contrast allergy), and allows for the acquisition of

a Department of Radiology, Division of Body Imaging, Hospital of the University of Pennsylvania, 3400 Spruce Street, Philadelphia, PA 19104, USA
b Department of Radiology, Hospital of the University of Pennsylvania, University of Pennsylvania School of Medicine, 3400 Spruce Street, Philadelphia, PA 19104, USA
* Corresponding author.
E-mail address: Drew.Torigian@uphs.upenn.edu

PET Clin 6 (2011) 37–54
doi:10.1016/j.cpet.2011.01.003

multiple image sequences that may each be useful to depict different inherent characteristics of disease processes. With the advent of stronger field strengths (1.5 and 3.0 T) and more advanced dedicated receiver coils, the improved soft-tissue contrast, spatial resolution, and signal-to-noise ratio (SNR) allow for greater lesion conspicuity.[6]

In addition to the inherent advantages of CT and MR imaging, the image acquisition protocol can be optimized to better detect certain disease processes. For CT, to best detect metastatic melanoma to the liver, a triple-phase hepatic imaging protocol is often implemented, because melanoma may be hypervascular. This protocol first starts with precontrast unenhanced image acquisition through the liver followed by postcontrast image acquisition obtained during the late arterial phase (25–35 second delay) and portal venous phase (50–75 second delay) of enhancement after the intravenous administration of iodinated contrast material administered via a power injector at a rate of 2.5 to 5 mL/s.[7] The late arterial phase is ideal for detecting hypervascular liver metastases because they recruit their primary blood supply from the hepatic arterial system, whereas the portal venous phase is optimal for detecting hypovascular or necrotic/cystic metastases. Because not all melanoma lesions are hypervascular, the implementation of this protocol maximizes the detection of metastatic melanoma to the liver.

For MR imaging, there are several ways to maximize detection of melanoma throughout the body. Standard pulse sequences used for MR imaging examination of the abdomen and pelvis include T1-weighted (T1-W) and T2-weighted (T2-W) sequences, which are obtained in axial and other orthogonal planes. In general, T1-W images (T1-WI) are useful for showing high signal intensity (SI) macroscopic fat, subacute hemorrhage, proteinaceous fluid, and other paramagnetic substances such as melanin. T1-WI are also useful for depicting low SI simple fluid and fibrous tissue, low SI iron deposition, intralesional microscopic lipid content, lymphadenopathy, and normal anatomy. The T1-W hyperintense SI when seen in melanoma is predominantly attributed to the presence of hemorrhage or melanin.[8] Although hyperintense T1-W SI can be helpful to detect and characterize metastatic melanoma lesions throughout the body, Premkumar and colleagues[9] found that only 26 (10%) of 261 metastatic melanoma lesions showed hyperintense T1-W SI. The most common MR imaging finding was a mass showing hypointense T1-W SI and hyperintense T2-W SI, which are nonspecific imaging characteristics that can be seen with other pathologic changes.[9] In general, T2-W images (T2-WI) are useful for showing high SI simple fluid, low SI fibrous tissue, and normal anatomy. Fat-suppressed T2-WI are useful for detecting and characterizing lesions within normal tissues, and for showing lymphadenopathy, muscle invasion by a disease process, cystic change or necrosis, fluid collections, tissue edema, and dilation or obstruction of fluid-containing hollow structures such as the ureters or biliary tree.[10]

Diffusion-weighted MR imaging (DWI) is a particular application of MR imaging that was first used clinically to detect cellular changes in the brain caused by acute cerebral infarction, but which has also been applied to detect, characterize, and monitor changes in tumors after therapeutic intervention, most often in the brain. However, it has been more difficult to use outside the brain, in part because of increased motion artifacts, low SNR, and long acquisition time.[11–13] The random translational diffusion of water molecules can be measured quantitatively with DWI.[14] DWI provides indirect information about water content, tissue structure, and the intracellular and extracellular spaces of tissue, and can be used to estimate tumor cellularity and to detect early changes in tumors after therapeutic intervention.[15] When cellular and subcellular compartmental membranes break down with apoptosis or necrosis, water molecules become less restricted to motion by diffusion.[14] However, when cellular swelling or increased tumor cellularity is encountered, water molecules become more restricted to motion by diffusion because of a reduction in the extracellular space, where most of the translational movement of water molecules occurs.[16] Through the quantitative assessment of such alterations in water diffusivity in different tissues, lesion detection and characterization may potentially be improved via this technology, which is currently a subject of active investigation. A study by Laurent and colleagues[17] showed a sensitivity and specificity for the detection of melanoma metastases by whole-body MR imaging of 82% and 97%, respectively. Addition of a DWI sequence to the standard MR imaging image acquisition protocol allowed for the detection of 14 additional malignant lesions (20%), with most lesions involving the bone marrow, liver, subcutaneous tissues, and peritoneum.[17] However, one of the greatest challenges to widespread clinical use of DWI in the body is the lack of standardization of image acquisition protocols and data analysis protocols across institutions.[12,18]

Numerous MR imaging contrast agents are available to improve lesion detection and characterization, particularly in the liver.[19] The 3 major classes of contrast agents used in clinical practice are extracellular agents, hepatobiliary agents, and combined agents. The feature common to all 3 of these agents is that they all result in T1 shortening, which is depicted as signal enhancement at T1-WI. Extracellular agents use gadolinium chelates, which enter various organs via their vascular supply and are freely redistributed into the extra-cellular interstitial space.[19] Gadolinium chelates have been in clinical use for the longest period among the different classes of contrast agents, and can be used for lesion detection, lesion characterization, and vascular assessment.[19] Whereas the iodine molecule is imaged directly on CT based on its ability to attenuate the radiograph beam, in MR imaging it is the indirect effect of the gadolinium atom on the T1 relaxation time of adjacent protons that is assessed rather than the molecule itself.[19] Gadolinium has an amplification effect in which many adjacent water molecules are relaxed by a single gadolinium atom.[19] As a result, MR imaging is orders of magnitude more sensitive to the effect of gadolinium than CT is to the effect of iodine.[20] Thus, subtle areas of contrast accumulation may be depicted with MR imaging that would not be detected with CT, lower doses of gadolinium are needed compared with iodinated contrast, and the blood pool remains visible for a longer period.[19] A typical imaging protocol using an extracellular contrast agent includes three-dimensional fat-suppressed T1-WI before and after the intravenous administration of contrast with dynamic imaging performed to improve lesion detection and characterization. As with triple-phase liver CT, dynamic imaging of the liver performed during arterial and portal venous phases of enhancement allows for improved lesion detection.

Hepatobiliary contrast agents are paramagnetic compounds that are taken up by functioning hepatocytes and excreted in bile.[19] In addition to the normal sequences obtained during the MR imaging examination, a delayed T1-W sequence is obtained during the hepatobiliary phase of enhancement from 10 to 120 minutes after intravenous administration, with the exact timing depending on the particular contrast agent used. Contrast agents in this class increase the T1 SI of normal hepatic parenchyma, bile ducts, and some hepatocyte-containing lesions during the hepatobiliary phase of enhancement.[21–23] Although these contrast agents are primarily used to distinguish hepatocellular from nonhepatocellular lesions, they may also be useful for improved detection of metastatic disease to the liver, which is an area of active investigation. The reason is that the increased T1-W SI of the normal background hepatic parenchyma (which takes up the contrast agent) and the low T1-W SI of hepatic metastases (as a result of lack of functioning hepatocytes) during the hepatobiliary phase of enhancement results in an increased contrast-to-noise ratio, thereby increasing lesion conspicuity.[24]

LIVER, GALLBLADDER, AND BILIARY TREE

The liver is a common site of melanoma metastases, and liver involvement has been associated with a particularly poor prognosis.[25] Recent expansion of therapeutic options for metastatic melanoma has led to increased interest in accurate detection and quantification of disease burden for prognosis, clinical trial stratification, and monitoring of therapy. As stated earlier, both CT and MR imaging are used in the detection of metastatic disease. US is useful to differentiate solid from cystic liver lesions, but is not so sensitive or specific as CT or MR imaging. Because metastases from melanoma are often hypervascular, many institutions empirically perform multiphasic CT through the liver. On unenhanced CT images, melanoma metastases are often low in attenuation unless complicated by hemorrhage, in which case they may have regions of higher attenuation. If the metastatic lesion is hypervascular, it often shows enhancement during the late arterial phase and becomes hypoattenuating to liver in the portal venous phase.[26] If the lesion is not hypervascular, it is depicted best on the portal venous phase as a low-attenuation lesion possibly with peripheral or rim enhancement. In a study performed by Blake and colleagues,[25] 48 of 57 hepatic metastatic melanoma lesions were seen on the arterial phase images, 49 on the portal venous phase images, and 30 on delayed phase images. Of 8 lesions (14%) overlooked on portal venous phase images, 6 were seen on unenhanced images and 6 were seen on arterial phase images, implying that more than 1 phase is needed for hepatic CT in patients with malignant melanoma.[25] However, CT is limited because of its association with radiation exposure and difficulty in characterizing lesions less than 1 cm in size.

MR imaging has emerged as the imaging modality of choice for detection and characterization of liver lesions.[26] MR imaging has a high lesion/liver contrast ratio and is not associated with a risk of radiation exposure.[26] The typical MR imaging protocol involves the use of T1-W and T2-W sequences along with dynamic postcontrast images obtained during late arterial, portal venous, and delayed phases of enhancement. Melanoma metastases may be variable in T1-W and T2-W SI but are usually hypointense to isointense on T1-WI and isointense to slightly hyperintensity on T2-WI relative to surrounding liver parenchyma, usually with SI similar to that of the spleen.[27] Metastases tend to lose signal on heavily T2-WI (echo time >160 ms) unlike hemangiomas and cysts, which typically have high SI.[28] The only exception is when a metastasis shows liquefactive necrosis resulting in a cystic appearance, which has been described in melanoma. Metastatic melanoma lesions may also show increased SI on T1-WI because of melanin or extracellular methemoglobin content. On DWI, these lesions appear hyperintense on low and high b-value images, with low SI seen on accompanying apparent diffusion coefficient (ADC) map images as a result of restricted diffusion. On dynamic contrast-enhanced images, the arterial phase enhancement may be uniform, peripheral/rim, or heterogeneous.[29] If the metastasis is more necrotic in nature, it may be better seen on the portal venous and delayed phases of enhancement. The peripheral washout sign is a specific but insensitive sign for hypervascular metastases that refers to contrast material preferentially washing out from the periphery of a lesion as seen on portal venous or more delayed phases of enhancement.[30] This sign is believed to be related to the degree of tumor vascularity, with increased peripheral vascularity (as a result of viable tumor) and decreased central vascularity (from necrosis or fibrosis).[30] Melanoma metastases typically appear hypointense relative to the liver on hepatobiliary phase T1-WI after the use of a hepatobiliary contrast agent. In a study performed by Muller-Horvat and colleagues,[28] MR imaging was superior to CT in the detection of small liver metastases and was able to detect more lesions than CT in 8 of 19 patients (42%). In 3 of 19 patients (16%), the diagnosis of liver metastases was established only by MR imaging.[28] The smallest lesion detected by MR imaging had a diameter of 3 mm, compared with 5 mm for CT.[28] MR imaging was particularly superior for the detection of small lesions (<1 cm), and additional studies comparing the usefulness of MR imaging with fluorodeoxyglucose (FDG)-PET/CT have found similar results.[5,17,28] See Figs. 1–3 for examples of liver metastasis.

The gallbladder is a well-known site of metastatic disease from malignant melanoma,

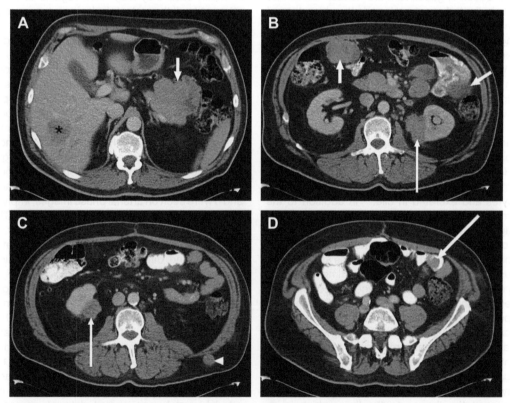

Fig. 1. Metastatic melanoma. (*A–D*) Axial contrast-enhanced CT images through abdomen and pelvis show multiple soft-tissue attenuation metastases involving liver (*), mesentery and omentum (*arrows*), kidneys (*long thin arrows*), subcutaneous fat (*arrowhead*), and small bowel (*long thick arrow*).

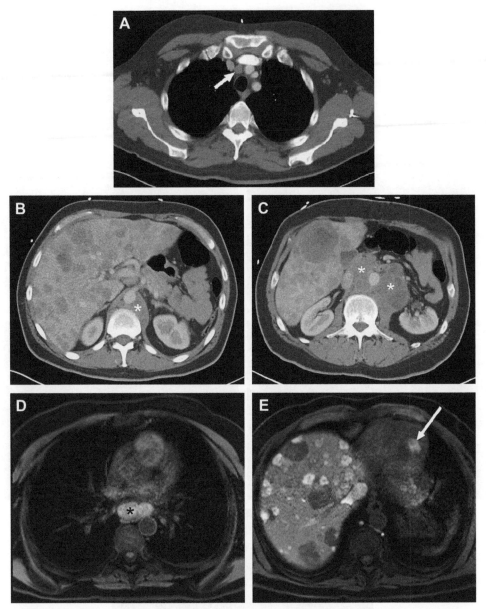

Fig. 2. Metastatic melanoma. (*A–C*) Axial contrast-enhanced CT images through chest and abdomen show multiple soft-tissue attenuation metastases involving pretracheal anterior mediastinal lymph node (*arrow*), retrocrural and retroperitoneal periaortic lymph nodes (***), and liver. (*D, E*) Axial fat-suppressed T1-WI through chest and abdomen reveal subcarinal lymphadenopathy (***), left ventricular cardiac metastasis (*arrow*), and multiple hepatic metastases, all with high SI as a result of melanin content. Hypointense lesions in (*E*) are caused by hepatic cysts.

accounting for 50% to 65% of metastatic tumors involving the gallbladder.[31,32] In a previous autopsy series of patients with malignant melanoma, it was reported that 15% of the cases featured metastases to the gallbladder.[31] On CT and US, metastatic melanoma can manifest as focal thickening of the gallbladder wall, a submucosal mass, or as single or multiple irregular polypoid intraluminal masses.[32,33] In cases of

involvement of the bile ducts, US and CT may show bile duct dilation and intraluminal mural masses.[34,35] On MR imaging, the SI on T1-WI again can be variable depending on the percentage of melanin-containing cells, necrosis, and hemorrhage. Metastatic lesions are often hyperintense on T2-WI and DWI, with the degree of hyperintensity depending on the amount of necrosis and cellularity. Postcontrast images

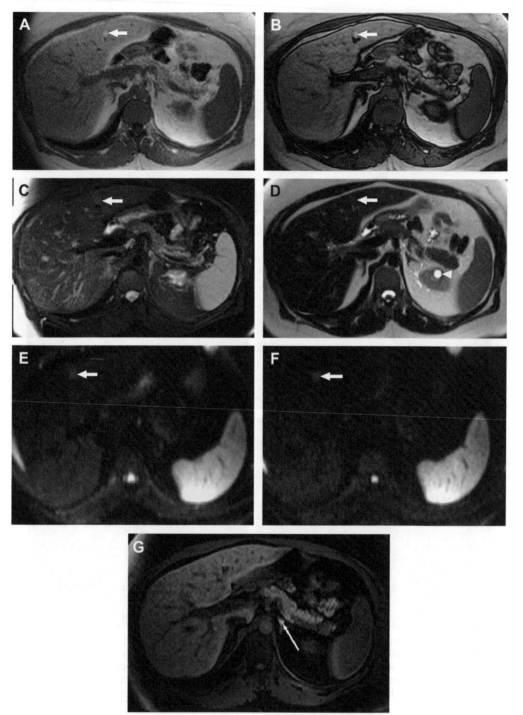

Fig. 3. Metastatic melanoma. (*A, B*) Axial T1-W in-phase (*A*) and opposed-phase (*B*) images through abdomen show lesion in lateral segment of liver (*arrow*) with high SI caused by melanin content but without loss of SI or surrounding black etching artifact on opposed-phase image, indicating lack of microscopic lipid content and lack of macroscopic fat content, respectively. Note black etching artifact at fat-water interfaces about abdominal organs on opposed-phase image. (*C, D*) Axial fat-suppressed T2-WI (*C*) shows lesion (*arrow*) with slightly hyperintense SI relative to liver but similar to that of spleen. Axial heavily T2-WI (*D*) reveals loss of SI of hepatic lesion (*arrow*), which makes cyst and hemangioma highly unlikely. Note very high SI of left renal cyst (*arrowhead*) and cerebrospinal fluid. (*E, F*) Axial DWI with low (*E*) and high (*F*) b values show high SI of lesion, which indicates restricted diffusion. Lesion SI on ADC map image (not shown) was low relative to liver, also in keeping with restricted diffusion. (*G*) Axial fat-suppressed T1-WI shows nodule (*long thin arrow*) within left adrenal gland as a result of metastasis. High SI in nodule is caused by increased melanin content.

contribute little to the characterization of melanotic lesions presenting with hyperintensity on precontrast T1-WI, and can even make their visualization difficult, because gadolinium may enhance normal mucosa and other normal structures.[9] In cases of suspected biliary tract involvement, the use of a heavily T2-W magnetic resonance cholangiopancreatography sequence may be useful to show intrahepatic or extrahepatic biliary ductal dilation with or without intraluminal filling defects. See **Fig. 4** for example of gallbladder metastasis.

SPLEEN

The spleen is a rare site for metastatic disease in patients who have cancer in general, with an incidence of 5% at autopsy.[36] However, one of the tumors most frequently implicated is malignant melanoma, with 30% of melanoma patients having splenic involvement at autopsy.[37] On CT, splenic metastases most often appear as ill-defined low-attenuation lesions. However, they can also appear as more well-defined cystic or solid masses. Melanoma can often result in cystic splenic metastases, believed to be related to rapid tumor growth resulting in autoinfarction, internal necrosis, or both.[38] Cystic or necrotic masses may show contrast enhancement at the periphery or within septa of the lesion.[39] On MR imaging, splenic metastases typically appear as hyperintense lesions on T2-WI and hypointense to isointense lesions on T1-WI.[40] Again, as in the liver, the degree of melanin content and presence of intralesional hemorrhage result in varying T1-W SI characteristics. In a study by Muller-Horvat and colleagues,[28] CT was able to detect 26 of 54 lesions (48%) in 6 of 9 patients (67%). In 2 of 9 patients (22%), MR imaging detected more lesions than CT and in 1 of 9 patients

(11%), lesions were detected only by MR imaging. See **Fig. 5** for example of splenic metastasis.

PANCREAS

In a study by Cubilla and Fitzgerald,[41] the leading primary tumors in 273 cases of pancreatic metastasis at autopsy were breast carcinoma (51 cases), lung carcinoma (49 cases), and melanoma (23 cases). In patients with malignant melanoma, the discovery of a pancreatic lesion either on CT or MR imaging can present a diagnostic dilemma to differentiate between a primary pancreatic neoplasm and a pancreatic metastasis. Certain coexisting factors can help the diagnostic imager favor one or the other. Multiplicity of tumors within the pancreas is relatively common in cases of metastases, whereas this is not characteristic of primary pancreatic carcinoma.[42] Coexisting metastases at sites that are not typically involved with pancreatic adenocarcinoma, such as the bone marrow, adrenal glands, and soft tissues, should also favor a diagnosis of pancreatic metastasis. Metastatic melanoma to the pancreas also has certain imaging features on both CT and MR imaging that are more characteristic of its extrapancreatic source. On contrast-enhanced CT, whereas pancreatic adenocarcinoma typically appears as a hypoenhancing mass, a large proportion of melanoma metastases show greater amounts of enhancement, and may be homogeneously or heterogeneously enhancing, either during the arterial or portal venous phase. Depending on the size of the lesion and the degree of necrosis and cystic degeneration, there may be a central poorly or nonenhancing component.

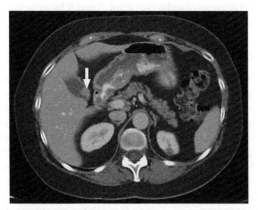

Fig. 4. Metastatic melanoma. Axial contrast-enhanced CT image through abdomen reveals enhancing soft-tissue attenuation polypoid mass (*arrow*) of gall-bladder caused by metastasis.

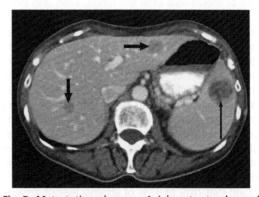

Fig. 5. Metastatic melanoma. Axial contrast-enhanced CT image through abdomen shows hypoattenuating hepatic lesions (*arrows*) and heterogeneous splenic lesion (*long arrow*) with continuous peripheral rim enhancement caused by metastases. Central hypoattenuating regions in splenic lesion are in keeping with necrosis.

Metastatic lesions may occur anywhere within the pancreas without predilection for any specific part. In a study by Klein and colleagues,[42] of 79 metastatic lesions involving the pancreas, 35.4% were located in the head, 22.8% in the body, and 35.4% in the tail. Because pancreatic adenocarcinoma is most often located in the pancreatic head, a lesion located in the body or tail in a patient with known melanoma makes the diagnosis of metastatic disease more likely. Problematic situations can arise either in a solitary pancreatic lesion with no other evidence of metastatic disease or in a pancreatic lesion discovered long after presumed successful treatment of the initial melanoma. Metastatic lesions to the pancreas have been found sometimes 5 to 6 years after presumed successful treatment.[42] Also, functioning and nonfunctioning islet cell tumors can have similar imaging features, and in these instances tissue diagnosis via percutaneous or endoscopic biopsy may be necessary.

On MR imaging, the imaging features of metastatic melanoma to the pancreas are similar to that of the liver. The lesion may show hypointense, isointense, or hyperintense SI on T1-WI depending on the degree of melanin and hemorrhage within the lesion. Lesions may be hyperenhancing on the arterial phase if the predominating feature is hypervascularity or may show more heterogeneous enhancement on the portal venous and delayed phases. The T2-WI SI characteristics also vary, with most lesions appearing slightly hyperintense to the background normal pancreatic parenchyma.

ADRENAL GLANDS

The adrenal glands are the fourth most common site of metastasis after the lungs, liver, and bone marrow.[43] Adrenal metastases from malignant melanoma are most often clinically and biochemically silent, which may contribute to their often large size at diagnosis.[43] In a study by Rajaratnam and Waugh[44] of 4 patients with adrenal metastases from malignant melanoma, the metastases ranged in size from 5 to 14 cm and the discovery of the lesions was made 3 to 6 years after the primary diagnosis, with no evidence of other metastatic lesions. Size and bilaterality of adrenal lesions are important predictors of metastatic disease. A study by Lockhart and colleagues[45] found that 78% to 87% of adrenal lesions smaller than 3 cm were benign and at least 90% of lesions larger than 3 cm were malignant. In a patient with known malignancy, benign adrenocortical adenoma is considered as a differential diagnostic consideration in addition to adrenal metastasis. Research studies have been performed to characterize adrenal lesions using both CT and MR imaging. On unenhanced CT, the mean attenuation method based on a threshold of 10 Hounsfield units (HU) is known to be useful for differentiating adenomas from metastases, and has a sensitivity of 71% for the diagnosis of adrenal adenoma.[46] If a lesion cannot be characterized as an adenoma on unenhanced CT, one option for further characterization is the use of a 15-minute delayed phase in addition to the portal venous phase of enhancement. Through acquisition of 15-minute delayed phase postcontrast images, the absolute percent washout of a lesion can be calculated using the following formula: $[(CT_{EE} - CT_{DE})/(CT_{EE} - CT_{UE})] \cdot 100\%$, where CT_{UE}, CT_{EE}, and CT_{DE} are the measured attenuation values in HU of the adrenal lesion using unenhanced, early enhanced, and delayed enhanced CT images, respectively.[47] An absolute percent washout of greater than 60% is characteristic of a benign adrenal adenoma, with sensitivity up to 97% and specificity near 100%.[47]

MR imaging can also be used to evaluate adrenal lesions. The use of chemical shift imaging allows detection of microscopic lipid within an adrenal lesion, which is characteristic of an adenoma. Presence of microscopic lipid in the lesion is depicted as a loss of SI within the lesion on the opposed-phase T1-WI when compared with the in-phase T1-WI. Adrenal metastases usually show low SI on T1-WI, although SI may be variably high depending on the amount of melanin and presence of hemorrhage, and high SI on T2-WI, with progressive enhancement after administration of contrast material.[48] The most important diagnostic feature again is the lack of signal loss on out-of-phase images. Both CT and MR imaging have been shown to be comparable in the detection of metastatic disease involving the adrenal glands. See **Figs. 3** and **6** for examples of adrenal gland metastasis.

KIDNEYS, URETERS, AND BLADDER

The kidneys, ureters, and bladder are rare sites of metastatic disease. Renal metastases from melanoma are usually found in cases of widespread metastatic disease. The most common metastases to the kidney are lung, breast, and gastric carcinomas, followed by melanoma.[49] Typically, renal metastases from melanoma are small (<1 cm), subcortical, multiple, and bilateral from hematogenous dissemination.[50] These metastases frequently invade through the renal capsule into the perinephric space.[51] In a study by Choyke and colleagues[52] of 27 patients with renal metastases, 2 of 4 patients with renal metastases from

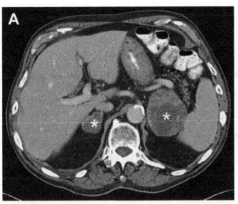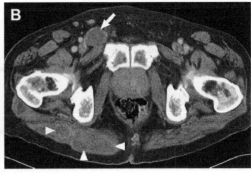

Fig. 6. Metastatic melanoma. (*A*) Axial contrast-enhanced CT image through abdomen shows heterogeneous enhancing adrenal masses (*) caused by metastases with areas of fluid attenuation necrosis or cystic change. (*B*) Axial contrast-enhanced CT image through pelvis reveals right inguinal lymphadenopathy (*arrow*) and subtle heterogeneous enhancing soft-tissue mass of right gluteal musculature (*arrowheads*) caused by metastatic disease.

metastatic melanoma showed bilateral involvement and 3 showed extension of tumor into the perinephric space. On CT and MR imaging, most lesions appear as circumscribed, enhancing, rounded masses, but truly infiltrative lesions are occasionally seen. Other imaging features such as an exophytic component, cystic or necrotic change, or hemorrhage can also be seen. There is a great deal of overlap between the imaging features of metastatic melanoma and primary renal cell carcinoma. On MR imaging, lesions may be hypointense or hyperintense on T1-WI, again depending on the presence of hemorrhage or melanin, and tend to be slightly hyperintense to the surrounding renal parenchyma on T2-WI depending on the degree of necrosis and cystic degeneration. Presence of microscopic lipid as detected on opposed-phase T1-WI favors a clear cell renal cell carcinoma, because lipid is not present in melanoma metastases. The degree of enhancement of melanoma metastases to the kidney is also variable, although some degree of enhancement either within or surrounding the lesion is invariably seen. Patients with a known extrarenal primary malignancy who present with a solitary renal lesion present a greater diagnostic challenge, because the possibility of a synchronous primary renal cancer must also be considered.[53] Because infiltrative growth is an uncommon manifestation of renal cortical tumors in general, a solitary infiltrative renal lesion in a patient with a history of melanoma most likely represents metastatic disease. However, tissue sampling is usually necessary in such cases. See **Fig. 1** for an example of kidney metastasis.

The true prevalence of hematogenous metastasis to the ureter is unknown, but is believed to be low.

Most lesions are asymptomatic and are found incidentally at autopsy. When present, symptoms are usually secondary to ureteral obstruction. Three patterns of metastatic involvement of the ureter have been described: infiltration of the periureteral soft tissues, transmural involvement of the ureteral wall, and submucosal nodules.[54] The first two may manifest as stricture formation with or without an associated mass. The third pattern is seen on imaging as 1 or more filling defects within the ureteral lumen. Adequate distention of the ureter must be achieved to detect intraluminal filling defects, and in the past, this was best achieved either with intravenous or retrograde urography. However, with the advent of CT, evaluation of the collection systems is now routinely performed with CT urography, which uses thin-section multiplanar image reconstruction during the delayed phase of enhancement typically after the intravenous administration of furosemide and saline to achieve maximal ureteral distention to detect intraluminal filling defects. The detection of an intraluminal filling defect in a patient with known advanced melanoma is highly suggestive of metastatic disease. There are currently ongoing studies regarding the usefulness of MR urography (MRU) as well, although this technique is limited by longer acquisition times and motion-related artifacts. As further advancements are made in regards to MR imaging technology and shorter scan times, MRU may play a larger role in evaluation of the urinary tract.

Metastatic melanoma to the bladder is uncommon. Most bladder lesions that are detected are caused by primary transitional cell carcinomas. As is the case with the remainder of the genitourinary system, metastatic disease to the bladder is usually seen in patients with advanced and widespread metastatic disease. Lesions may be mucosal or submucosal in location, and may be smooth and well-circumscribed or irregular and infiltrative. Cystoscopy and biopsy may be necessary for a definitive diagnosis.

GASTROINTESTINAL TRACT

Malignant melanoma is 1 of the most common tumors to metastasize to the gastrointestinal (GI) tract, represents about one-third of all metastatic disease to the GI tract, and is found in 58% of postmortem specimens in patients with melanoma.[55,56] Within the GI tract, the small bowel is the most common site of metastatic involvement.[57] Although metastatic melanoma to the GI tract is associated with a poor prognosis when treatment involves incomplete surgical resection, several surgical outcome studies have showed prolonged survival in selected patients after complete resection of small bowel metastases. Therefore, detection of metastatic disease to the GI tract can play a significant role in patient management. Antemortem diagnosis of disease involving the GI tact is made in only 1.5% to 4.4% of all patients with melanoma, thus showing the difficulty of detection and limitations of structural imaging studies.[55,58] The 2 most commonly used radiologic studies for evaluating the GI tract are fluoroscopic barium studies and contrast-enhanced CT. Although barium studies provide more detail regarding mucosal disease, CT (particularly when oral contrast material is administered) offers the advantages of better visualization of bowel loops and detection of extraluminal disease, whether located in the adjacent mesentery or at additional sites in the body.[59] The sensitivity of detection of metastases in the small bowel has been shown to be 58% and 66% for fluoroscopic small bowel follow-through examination and contrast-enhanced CT, respectively.[60] The use of CT enteroclysis, which allows for greater small bowel distention and opacification via thin-section multiplanar reconstructions and administration of a large volume of dilute oral contrast material, can improve the detection of more subtle lesions.

Bender and colleagues[60] defined 4 different morphologic patterns of metastatic involvement of the small bowel on barium examination and CT: (1) cavitary (a circumferential or infiltrating mass with a central collection of contrast or air contiguous with adjacent bowel and irregular inner margins); (2) infiltrative (a mass with a central collection of contrast or air communicating with adjacent bowel and with a fixed decrease in caliber compared with normal bowel loops

[including apple core lesions]); (3) exoenteric (a mass that involves more than 1 bowel loop with the bulk of the lesion in an extraluminal or mesenteric location); or (4) polypoid (a smooth or fungating intraluminal mass with or without ulceration, the former often referred to as a target lesion). On examination of the pathologic specimens of 32 cases, 20 (63%) involved polypoid lesions, 3 (9%) showed a target lesion appearance, 8 (25%) showed a cavitary mass, and 5 (16%) showed an infiltrative lesion. Overall, lesions were distributed evenly between the jejunum and ileum. An additional finding that can be seen on both barium studies and CT is that of an intussusception, where a visualized or occult metastatic lesion involving the bowel can serve as a lead point. Therefore, whenever an intussusception is encountered in a patient with known melanoma, particularly in adults, strong consideration should be given for an underlying metastatic lesion.

MR imaging has limited usefulness in the evaluation of the GI tract because of the higher cost of examination, longer examination time (with associated increased motion artifacts on some MR pulse sequences related to bowel peristalsis), lower spatial resolution, and variability in examination quality (related to patient cooperation and breath-holding ability) compared with CT.[61] Current indications for MR imaging of the small bowel include patients with Crohn disease (in particular for optimal detection and delineation of sinus and fistulous tracts in the perirectal/perianal region), patients in whom radiation exposure is a concern, patients who cannot undergo CT, and patients with low-grade small bowel obstruction.[61] There is promise for the future usefulness of MR imaging of the GI tract given its inherent advantages (lack of ionizing radiation, superior soft-tissue contrast resolution) and the use of spasmolytic drugs. Much research is under way with regards to MR enterography and MR enteroclysis in the evaluation of bowel disease.

An advantage of MR imaging over CT for the detection of small bowel masses is the ability of MR imaging to generate images with different gradations of intraluminal contrast agents. At CT, hyperenhancing masses are well depicted when negative enteric contrast material is administered; however, some masses are isoattenuating relative to the bowel wall, and in areas with suboptimal distention, such masses may be difficult to detect. The alternative use of a positive enteric contrast agent at CT may mask the enhancement of hyperenhancing masses.[61] The use of biphasic enteric contrast agents at MR imaging (which have low T1-W and high T2-W SI) may help overcome this limitation. On T2-WI, small bowel masses show lower SI than intraluminal fluid, a characteristic that may help identify masses that do not show substantial enhancement after intravenous contrast material is administered.[61] A pitfall of T2-WI is that artifactual low SI voids can be seen in the lumen as a result of peristalsis and fluid motion, although these tend to be inconstant in appearance over the time of the imaging examination. Heavily T2-W fast spin echo sequences are generally more susceptible to this pitfall compared with balanced steady state free precession sequences, and spasmolytics may help to reduce such artifacts. Overall, there is a paucity of data regarding the sensitivity of MR imaging for the detection of small bowel masses.[61] See **Figs. 1** and **7** for examples of GI tract metastasis.

LYMPH NODES AND MESENTERY

Both CT and MR imaging have usefulness in the detection of lymphadenopathy throughout the body. Muller-Horvat and colleagues[28] compared the usefulness of whole-body MR imaging and CT in patients with malignant melanoma, and found that MR imaging and CT detected the same number of metastatic lymph nodes in the cervical, axillary, inguinal, mesentery, and pelvic/iliac regions. In the mediastinal region, MR imaging was able to detect 6 suspicious lymph nodes, whereas CT was able to detect only 3 of them. In the hilar region, CT found 11 suspicious lymph nodes with a mean diameter of 22 ± 10 mm, whereas MR imaging was able to detect 8. Both CT and MR imaging can detect enlarged lymph nodes well, where lymph nodes that measure greater than 1 cm in short-axis dimension are generally

considered as pathologic. Fat-suppressed T2-WI are frequently useful for the detection of lymph nodes, which are depicted as hyperintense soft-tissue foci in the expected locations of lymph node chains, although precontrast and postcontrast T1-WI are also useful. However, the major limitation of CT, MR imaging, and all other structural imaging techniques for evaluation of the lymph nodes is their suboptimal sensitivity and specificity for detection and characterization of metastatic disease in this location. This finding is a result of the observations that metastatic disease may be found in normal size lymph nodes and that enlargement of lymph nodes may alternatively be secondary to nonneoplastic causes such as infection or noninfectious inflammation. As a result, there has been great emphasis on FDG-PET/CT to improve the detection of metastatic disease within lymph nodes and to improve the characterization of lymphadenopathy as neoplastic or nonneoplastic.

There is also ongoing research with MR imaging contrast agents to perform MR lymphography, where superparamagnetic iron oxide (SPIO) particles are the most widely studied agent. Intravenously injected SPIO particles pass through the vascular endothelium into the interstitium of tissues, and are then taken up in normally functioning lymph nodes by cells of the reticuloendothelial system. As a result, normal lymph nodes generally show an SI decrease on T2*-WI and T2-WI because of effects of increased magnetic susceptibility and T2 shortening, whereas metastatic lymph nodes do not show reduced SI, potentially allowing for improved differentiation between benign and malignant lymph nodes.[62]

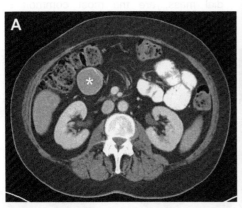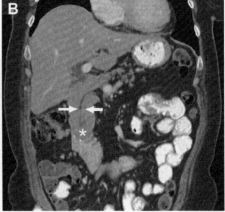

Fig. 7. Metastatic melanoma. (*A*) Axial contrast-enhanced CT image through abdomen shows soft-tissue attenuation mass (*) within loop of small bowel caused by metastasis. (*B*) Coronal reconstructed CT image shows tubular soft tissue within small bowel lumen superior and adjacent to metastasis (*), which contains thin curvilinear low-attenuation mesenteric fat and thin curvilinear high attenuation enhancing mesenteric vessel (*between arrows*), in keeping with small bowel intussusception.

Both CT and MR imaging are also useful in detecting metastatic involvement of the mesentery, and may show enhancing mesenteric masses with or without involvement of the small bowel. T1-WI generally depict lymphadenopathy as low SI masses, whereas on fat-suppressed T2-WI and DWI, they generally appear as hyperintense masses. See **Figs. 1, 2**, and **6** for examples of lymph node and mesenteric metastasis.

LUNGS AND HEART

The lung is the most frequently affected organ by metastatic melanoma at autopsy.[37] Chest radiography and thoracic CT form the mainstay of imaging of pulmonary metastases, and CT is superior to MR imaging for the detection of pulmonary metastases. The higher spatial resolution, higher lesion/background contrast ratio in the lungs, and faster scan time of CT are qualities that are ideal for lung imaging. However, respiratory motion-related artifacts and susceptibility artifacts created by air within the lung make MR imaging a markedly suboptimal modality for oncologic pulmonary imaging. Muller-Horvat and colleagues[28] found that whole-body CT detected more lung metastases than whole-body MR imaging. In 2 of 20 patients (10%) lung metastases were depicted by CT with a mean diameter of 5 ± 1 mm, CT detected more lung metastases than MR imaging in 6 of 20 patients (30%), and 24% of 199 nodules detected by CT were not visible on MR imaging. Therefore, CT is currently considered as the gold standard for detection of pulmonary nodules.

The imaging features of pulmonary metastatic disease from melanoma are variable, and may include solitary or multiple nodules (≤3 cm) or masses (>3 cm), a miliary nodular interstitial pattern, lymphangitic carcinomatosis (as manifested by smooth or nodular interlobular septal thickening that is typically asymmetric), or an endotracheal or endobronchial mass that may be associated with postobstructive pneumonia or atelectasis. Less common imaging findings include a cavitary nodule or nodule with surrounding ground glass attenuation as a result of perilesional hemorrhage.[63] Because the spread of melanoma is most often hematogenous, the lower lobes are most commonly affected. In a study by Miyake and colleagues,[63] 5 of 9 patients with pulmonary melanoma metastases had a solitary pulmonary nodule and 4 had multiple nodules. The most common imaging feature was a solid nodule with well-defined smooth margins. Fifty percent of patients with pulmonary nodules caused by metastatic melanoma also have enlarged mediastinal and hilar lymph nodes. Because pulmonary nodules can be seen in a variety of disease entities ranging from infectious to noninfectious inflammatory to neoplastic, tissue diagnosis or short-term follow-up imaging may be necessary if no other sites of metastatic melanoma are found. See **Fig. 8** for an example of pulmonary metastasis.

Metastatic disease to the heart is more common than primary cardiac malignancy. In 30% to 50% of patients with melanoma, cardiac metastases are found at autopsy, whereas only 2% are discovered ante mortem.[64] Melanomas have the highest prevalence of cardiac metastases of any neoplasm.[65] All cardiac structures (endocardium, myocardium, and epicardium) may be involved, although the epicardium is the site most commonly affected by metastases.[66,67] The left ventricular free wall and the ventricular septum, the portions of the heart with the greatest myocardial mass, are the most common sites for

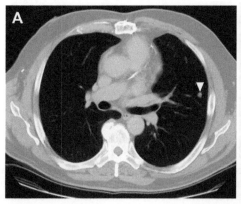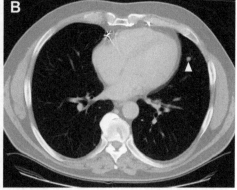

Fig. 8. Metastatic melanoma. (*A, B*) Axial contrast-enhanced CT images through chest reveal two subcentimeter nodules (*arrowheads*) in left upper lobe and lingula caused by metastases.

myocardial lesions. Endocardial metastases manifest as intracavitary lesions, can block inflow to the heart or outflow from a ventricular cavity, and can lead to tumor embolism to various organs of the body.[68]

The 4 pathways of cardiac invasion are retrograde lymphatic extension, hematogenous spread, direct contiguous extension, and transvenous extension.[69] Generally, melanoma is disseminated by means of hematogenous spread to the myocardium and epicardium via the coronary arteries or, less frequently, from the vena cavae.[70] Because microcirculation in the lungs and liver filters out most cancerous cells, these cells rarely reach the coronary arteries. Thus, hematogenous metastases to the heart and pericardium are often associated with hematogenous metastases to other organs.[71]

Many studies have shown the effectiveness of MR imaging for detection and definition of the anatomy of cardiac and pericardiac masses.[72] Cardiac tumors typically have low SI on T1-WI and high SI on T2-WI relative to muscle, and typically show enhancement.[73,74] Melanoma metastases again may show hyperintense T1-W SI as a result of melanin or hemorrhagic content. On CT, a nonspecific mass of the cardiac wall may be visualized. See **Fig. 2** for an example of cardiac metastasis.

BONE AND BONE MARROW

Bone marrow metastases occur in 11% to 17% of patients with melanoma with widespread metastatic disease.[28] Hematogenously seeded tumor cells accumulate in the intramedullary compartment, leading to replacement of the normal fatty or hematopoietic marrow and tumor cell proliferation before a reactive osteoblastic or osteoclastic response occurs. This is the reason that numerous studies have shown the extremely high sensitivity and specificity of MR imaging in the early detection of bone metastases when compared with skeletal scintigraphy, conventional radiography, and CT. These latter modalities depict the reactive changes in the cortical or medullary bone from tumor involvement rather than showing tumor infiltration of the bone marrow directly, whereas MR imaging allows for direct visualization of the bone marrow with high anatomic and spatial resolution.[75,76] In comparing whole-body MR imaging versus CT, Muller-Horvat and colleagues[28] found that MR imaging detected 132 lesions in 13 of 41 patients, whereas CT detected only 23 of 132 lesions (17%) in 5 of 13 patients. In 8 of 13 patients, 109 of 132 lesions (83%) were detected only by MR imaging, and in 4 of 13 patients, MR imaging was able to detect more lesions than CT. The combination of a T1-WI and fat-suppressed T2-WI has proved most accurate in the detection of malignant bone lesions.[77] On T1-WI, tumor is typically identified as areas of nonlipid-containing tissue within the normal lipid-containing bone marrow, the latter of which is normally hyperintense because of a high percentage of fat content, resulting in an isointense or hypointense SI of metastases relative to skeletal muscle. On fat-suppressed T2-WI, neoplastic lesions are readily detected by virtue of the hyperintense SI caused by an increased content of water within the tumor cells.[77] In severely sclerotic metastases, lesions may show hypointense T1-W and T2-W SI. If there is a high content of melanin within the osseous metastases, the paramagnetic effects causing hyperintense T1-W SI may make detection difficult on T1-WI alone because of the normally hyperintense SI of the background marrow. In these cases, lesions are more readily visible on fat-suppressed T2-WI. Lesion enhancement after intravenous contrast administration is markedly variable and can be homogeneous, heterogeneous, or absent. Gadolinium-based contrast does improve detection of soft-tissue tumor extension and, in cases of vertebral involvement, detection of leptomeningeal involvement. In cases of vertebral metastatic disease, MR imaging offers the additional advantage of detailed visualization of the spinal canal and spinal cord, providing an accurate means to assess for spinal cord compression.

When visualized on CT, melanoma metastases to the osseous structures are most often depicted as osteolytic lesions. The axial skeleton is most frequently affected because it contains most of the metabolically active bone marrow elements in adults. In cases of diffuse bone marrow infiltration, inhomogeneous osteopenia may be detected, which may be nonspecific in cause. CT offers the advantage of depiction of the degree of bone destruction, and can be useful for the assessment of cortical bone stability and fracture risk.[78,79] Both CT and MR imaging can detect soft-tissue extension of tumor into adjacent structures, although MR imaging is more sensitive given its higher contrast resolution. See **Figs. 9** and **10** for examples of osseous metastasis.

SOFT TISSUES

Despite the finding that the soft tissues comprise 55% of our body mass, hematogenous metastases to the soft tissues are rare.[80] Many theories have been postulated as to why metastases to the soft tissues are rare. These theories include changes in pH, accumulation of metabolites, and the local temperature at soft-tissue

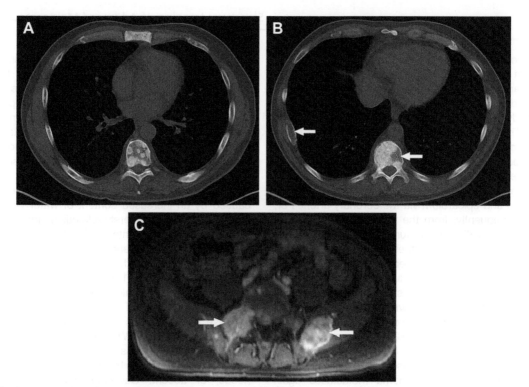

Fig. 9. Metastatic melanoma. (*A, B*) Axial unenhanced CT images through chest show multiple sclerotic lesions within sternum and thoracic spine as well as lytic lesions within thoracic spine and right rib (*arrows*) caused by osseous metastatic disease. (*C*) Axial fat-suppressed contrast-enhanced T1-WI through pelvis shows heterogeneously enhancing masses (*arrows*) involving sacrum and left iliac bone caused by bone marrow metastases.

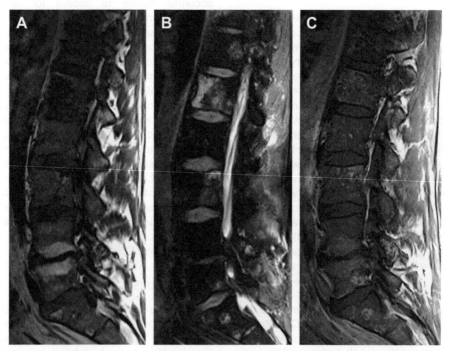

Fig. 10. Metastatic melanoma. (*A–C*) Sagittal T1-W (*A*), fat-suppressed T2-W (*B*), and contrast-enhanced T1-W (*C*) images through lumbar spine reveal multiple lesions in bone marrow with low SI on T1-WI, heterogeneously increased SI on T2-WI, and heterogeneous enhancement in keeping with bone marrow metastases. Endplate SI changes and disc space narrowing at L4 to 5 disc space level are caused by degenerative disease.

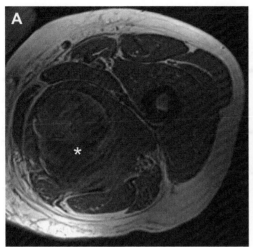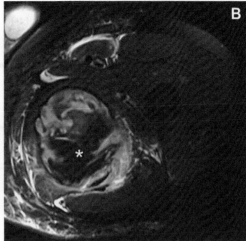

Fig. 11. Metastatic melanoma. (*A, B*) Axial T1-W (*A*) and fat-suppressed T2-W (*B*) images through thigh show large mass (*) within medial thigh musculature with heterogeneous SI caused by intratumoral hemorrhage. Curvilinear high SI areas in surrounding muscles and subcutaneous fat on T2-WI are caused by edema.

sites.[81] In addition, organs with a high predisposition for metastatic carcinomas, such as the liver or lung, are rich in capillary vessels and have a constant blood flow, whereas in soft tissues such as skeletal muscle, the blood flow is variable, is influenced by adrenergic receptors, and is subject to variations in tissue pressure affecting tumor implantation.[82] Of tumors that have been found to metastasize to the soft tissues, including muscle, subcutaneous fat, and skin, melanoma is one of the most common. In a study by Plaza and colleagues[53] of 118 cases of soft-tissue metastases, 20 were secondary to metastatic melanoma. In general, when metastases are seen in the soft tissues, there are coexisting sites of metastatic disease. Both CT and MR imaging can detect soft-tissue metastases, where MR imaging is more sensitive because of its superior contrast resolution. Horvat-Muller and colleagues[28] found that MR imaging detected 61 subcutaneous metastases in 12 of 41 patients, whereas CT detected 39 of 61 lesions (64%) in 4 of 12 patients. In 6 of 12 patients, MR imaging was able to detect more lesions than CT, and in 2 of 12 patients (17%) lesions were detected only by MR imaging. Eleven muscle metastases were detected by MR imaging in 8 of 41 patients, and of these 11 lesions, 7 were seen only by MR imaging.

On MR imaging, soft-tissue melanoma metastases may have variable SI on T1-WI, are typically hyperintense on fat-suppressed T2-WI relative to skeletal muscle, and show enhancement. In a patient with known melanoma, a soft-tissue lesion showing hyperintense T1-W SI and no macroscopic fat content is highly suspicious for metastatic disease. On CT, lesions within the subcutaneous fat are readily detected because of the high lesion contrast against the background of low-attenuation fat. Lesions within other soft tissues such as muscle are more difficult to detect because of the poor soft-tissue contrast resolution when compared with that of MR imaging. In a patient with known melanoma, extra attention should be paid to inspection of the soft tissues on both CT and MR imaging because of the increased prevalence of metastases in these locations and their subtle appearance. Laurent and colleagues[17] found that addition of DWI allowed for the improved detection of subcutaneous metastases as a result of improved contrast between the lesion and the surrounding tissues. See **Figs. 1, 6**, and **11** for examples of soft-tissue metastasis.

SUMMARY

The incidence and prevalence of metastatic melanoma continue to increase worldwide. Because the prognosis and treatment of melanoma greatly depend on the extent of disease at the time of diagnosis and after treatment, it is essential to have diagnostic tests that can accurately detect and characterize sites of metastatic disease. Both CT and MR imaging are widely used modalities to determine the extent of disease. Understanding the strengths and weaknesses of each modality in general and with regards to individual organ systems is essential to accurately assess for metastatic disease. Through implementation of tailored CT image acquisition protocols, novel MR imaging contrast agents, and advanced MR imaging pulse sequences such as DWI, the diagnostic imager can increase the diagnostic performance of lesion detection and characterization through structural imaging. As new technological advances continue to become available in structural and molecular imaging, diagnostic imagers will likely be able to diagnose advanced melanoma in earlier stages with improved sensitivity and specificity.

REFERENCES

1. Jemal A, Siegel R, Ward E, et al. Cancer statistics, 2009. CA Cancer J Clin 2009;59(4):225–49.
2. Rigel DS. Trends in dermatology: melanoma incidence. Arch Dermatol 2010;146(3):318.
3. Balch CM, Soong SJ, Gershenwald JE, et al. Prognostic factors analysis of 17,600 melanoma patients: validation of the American Joint Committee on Cancer melanoma staging system. J Clin Oncol 2001;19(16):3622–34.
4. Balch CM, Gershenwald JE, Soong SJ, et al. Final version of 2009 AJCC melanoma staging and classification. J Clin Oncol 2009;27(36):6199–206.
5. Pfannenberg C, Aschoff P, Schanz S, et al. Prospective comparison of 18F-fluorodeoxyglucose positron emission tomography/computed tomography and whole-body magnetic resonance imaging in staging of advanced malignant melanoma. Eur J Cancer 2007;43(3):557–64.
6. Choi JY, Kim MJ, Chung YE, et al. Abdominal applications of 3.0-T MR imaging: comparative review versus a 1.5-T system. Radiographics 2008; 28(4):e30.
7. Boll DT, Merkle EM. Diffuse liver disease: strategies for hepatic CT and MR imaging. Radiographics 2009;29(6):1591–614.
8. Premkumar A, Marincola F, Taubenberger J, et al. Metastatic melanoma: correlation of MRI characteristics and histopathology. J Magn Reson Imaging 1996;6(1):190–4.
9. Premkumar A, Sanders L, Marincola F, et al. Visceral metastases from melanoma: findings on MR imaging. AJR Am J Roentgenol 1992;158(2):293–8.
10. Low RN, Semelka RC, Worawattanakul S, et al. Extrahepatic abdominal imaging in patients with malignancy: comparison of MR imaging and helical CT, with subsequent surgical correlation. Radiology 1999;210(3):625–32.
11. Akisik FM, Sandrasegaran K, Aisen AM, et al. Abdominal MR imaging at 3.0 T. Radiographics 2007;27(5):1433–44 [discussion: 62–4].
12. Koh DM, Collins DJ. Diffusion-weighted MRI in the body: applications and challenges in oncology. AJR Am J Roentgenol 2007;188(6):1622–35.
13. Le Bihan D, Mangin JF, Poupon C, et al. Diffusion tensor imaging: concepts and applications. J Magn Reson Imaging 2001;13(4):534–46.
14. Le Bihan D, Poupon C, Amadon A, et al. Artifacts and pitfalls in diffusion MRI. J Magn Reson Imaging 2006;24(3):478–88.
15. Chenevert TL, Meyer CR, Moffat BA, et al. Diffusion MRI: a new strategy for assessment of cancer therapeutic efficacy. Mol Imaging 2002;1(4):336–43.
16. Mascalchi M, Filippi M, Floris R, et al. Diffusion-weighted MR of the brain: methodology and clinical application. Radiol Med 2005;109(3):155–97.
17. Laurent V, Trausch G, Bruot O, et al. Comparative study of two whole-body imaging techniques in the case of melanoma metastases: advantages of multi-contrast MRI examination including a diffusion-weighted sequence in comparison with PET-CT. Eur J Radiol 2010;75(3):376–83.
18. Lichy MP, Aschoff P, Plathow C, et al. Tumor detection by diffusion-weighted MRI and ADC-mapping–initial clinical experiences in comparison to PET-CT. Invest Radiol 2007;42(9):605–13.
19. Gandhi SN, Brown MA, Wong JG, et al. MR contrast agents for liver imaging: what, when, how. Radiographics 2006;26(6):1621–36.
20. Balci NC, Semelka RC. Contrast agents for MR imaging of the liver. Radiol Clin North Am 2005; 43(5):887–98, viii.
21. Giovagnoni A, Paci E. Liver. III: Gadolinium-based hepatobiliary contrast agents (Gd-EOB-DTPA and Gd-BOPTA/Dimeg). Magn Reson Imaging Clin N Am 1996;4(1):61–72.
22. Lim KO, Stark DD, Leese PT, et al. Hepatobiliary MR imaging: first human experience with MnDPDP. Radiology 1991;178(1):79–82.
23. Reimer P, Schneider G, Schima W. Hepatobiliary contrast agents for contrast-enhanced MRI of the liver: properties, clinical development and applications. Eur Radiol 2004;14(4):559–78.
24. Seale MK, Catalano OA, Saini S, et al. Hepatobiliary-specific MR contrast agents: role in imaging the liver and biliary tree. Radiographics 2009;29(6):1725–48.
25. Blake SP, Weisinger K, Atkins MB, et al. Liver metastases from melanoma: detection with multiphasic contrast-enhanced CT. Radiology 1999;213(1):92–6.
26. Namasivayam S, Salman K, Mittal PK, et al. Hypervascular hepatic focal lesions: spectrum of imaging features. Curr Probl Diagn Radiol 2007; 36(3):107–23.
27. Namasivayam S, Martin DR, Saini S. Imaging of liver metastases: MRI. Cancer Imaging 2007;7:2–9.
28. Muller-Horvat C, Radny P, Eigentler TK, et al. Prospective comparison of the impact on treatment decisions of whole-body magnetic resonance imaging and computed tomography in patients with metastatic malignant melanoma. Eur J Cancer 2006;42(3):342–50.

29. Silva AC, Evans JM, McCullough AE, et al. MR imaging of hypervascular liver masses: a review of current techniques. Radiographics 2009;29(2):385–402.

30. Mahfouz AE, Hamm B, Wolf KJ. Peripheral washout: a sign of malignancy on dynamic gadolinium enhanced MR images of focal liver lesions. Radiology 1994;190(1):49–52.

31. Dasgupta T, Brasfield R. Metastatic melanoma: a clinico-pathological study. Cancer 1964;10:1323–39.

32. Medina V, Darnell A, Bejarano N, et al. Primary biliary tract malignant melanoma: US, CT, and MR findings. Abdom Imaging 2003;28(6):842–6.

33. Takayama Y, Asayama Y, Yoshimitsu K, et al. Metastatic melanoma of the gallbladder. Comput Med Imaging Graph 2007;31(6):469–71.

34. Deugnier Y, Turlin B, Lehry D, et al. Malignant melanoma of the hepatic and common bile ducts. A case report and review of the literature. Arch Pathol Lab Med 1991;115(9):915–7.

35. Gates J, Kane RA, Hartnell GG. Primary biliary tract malignant melanoma. Abdom Imaging 1996;21(5):453–5.

36. King DM. Imaging of metastatic melanoma. Cancer Imaging 2006;6:204–8.

37. Patel JK, Didolkar MS, Pickren JW, et al. Metastatic pattern of malignant melanoma. A study of 216 autopsy cases. Am J Surg 1978;135(6):807–10.

38. Urrutia M, Mergo PJ, Ros LH, et al. Cystic masses of the spleen: radiologic-pathologic correlation. Radiographics 1996;16(1):107–29.

39. Silverman PM, Heaston DK, Korobkin M, et al. Computed tomography in the detection of abdominal metastases from malignant melanoma. Invest Radiol 1984;19(4):309–12.

40. Elsayes KM, Narra VR, Mukundan G, et al. MR imaging of the spleen: spectrum of abnormalities. Radiographics 2005;25(4):967–82.

41. Cubilla A, Fitzgerald P. Surgical pathology of tumors of the exocrine pancreas. Baltimore (MD): Williams & Wilkins; 1980. p. 159–93.

42. Klein KA, Stephens DH, Welch TJ. CT characteristics of metastatic disease of the pancreas. Radiographics 1998;18(2):369–78.

43. Wansaicheong G, Goh J. Adrenal metastases. Omaha (NE): WebMD LLC; 2002. Available from: http://www.emedicine.com/radio/TOPIC17.HTM. Accessed January 31, 2011.

44. Rajaratnam A, Waugh J. Adrenal metastases of malignant melanoma: characteristic computed tomography appearances. Australas Radiol 2005;49(4):325–9.

45. Lockhart ME, Smith JK, Kenney PJ. Imaging of adrenal masses. Eur J Radiol 2002;41(2):95–112.

46. Boland GW, Lee MJ, Gazelle GS, et al. Characterization of adrenal masses using unenhanced CT: an analysis of the CT literature. AJR Am J Roentgenol 1998;171(1):201–4.

47. Park BK, Kim CK, Kim B, et al. Comparison of delayed enhanced CT and chemical shift MR for evaluating hyperattenuating incidental adrenal masses. Radiology 2007;243(3):760–5.

40. Elsayes KM, Mukundan G, Narra VR, et al. Adrenal masses: MR imaging features with pathologic correlation. Radiographics 2004;24(Suppl 1):S73–86.

49. Bailey JE, Roubidoux MA, Dunnick NR. Secondary renal neoplasms. Abdom Imaging 1998;23(3):266–74.

50. Stein BS, Kendall AR. Malignant melanoma of the genitourinary tract. J Urol 1984;132(5):859–68.

51. Shimko MS, Jacobs SC, Phelan MW. Renal metastasis of malignant melanoma with unknown primary. Urology 2007;69(2):384, e9–10.

52. Choyke PL, White EM, Zeman RK, et al. Renal metastases: clinicopathologic and radiologic correlation. Radiology 1987;162(2):359–63.

53. Plaza JA, Perez-Montiel D, Mayerson J, et al. Metastases to soft tissue: a review of 118 cases over a 30-year period. Cancer 2008;112(1):193–203.

54. Winalski CS, Lipman JC, Tumeh SS. Ureteral neoplasms. Radiographics 1990;10(2):271–83.

55. Dasgupta TK, Brasfield RD. Metastatic melanoma of the gastrointestinal tract. Arch Surg 1964;88:969–73.

56. Washington K, McDonagh D. Secondary tumors of the gastrointestinal tract: surgical pathologic findings and comparison with autopsy survey. Mod Pathol 1995;8(4):427–33.

57. Blecker D, Abraham S, Furth EE, et al. Melanoma in the gastrointestinal tract. Am J Gastroenterol 1999;94(12):3427–33.

58. Reintgen DS, Thompson W, Garbutt J, et al. Radiologic, endoscopic, and surgical considerations of melanoma metastatic to the gastrointestinal tract. Surgery 1984;95(6):635–9.

59. Lens M, Bataille V, Krivokapic Z. Melanoma of the small intestine. Lancet Oncol 2009;10(5):516–21.

60. Bender GN, Maglinte DD, McLarney JH, et al. Malignant melanoma: patterns of metastasis to the small bowel, reliability of imaging studies, and clinical relevance. Am J Gastroenterol 2001;96(8):2392–400.

61. Fidler JL, Guimaraes L, Einstein DM. MR imaging of the small bowel. Radiographics 2009;29(6):1811–25.

62. Mack MG, Balzer JO, Straub R, et al. Superparamagnetic iron oxide-enhanced MR imaging of head and neck lymph nodes. Radiology 2002;222(1):239–44.

63. Miyake M, Tateishi U, Maeda T, et al. Pulmonary involvement of malignant melanoma: thin-section CT findings with pathologic correlation. Radiat Med 2005;23(7):497–503.

64. van Beek EJ, Stolpen AH, Khanna G, et al. CT and MRI of pericardial and cardiac neoplastic disease. Cancer Imaging 2007;7:19–26.

65. Glancy DL, Roberts WC. The heart in malignant melanoma. A study of 70 autopsy cases. Am J Cardiol 1968;21(4):555–71.

66. Klatt EC, Heitz DR. Cardiac metastases. Cancer 1990;65(6):1456–9.

67. Lam KY, Dickens P, Chan AC. Tumors of the heart. A 20-year experience with a review of 12,485 consecutive autopsies. Arch Pathol Lab Med 1993;117(10): 1027–31.

68. Roberts WC. Primary and secondary neoplasms of the heart. Am J Cardiol 1997;80(5):671–82.

69. Schoen FJ, Berger BM, Guerina NG. Cardiac effects of noncardiac neoplasms. Cardiol Clin 1984;2(4): 657–70.

70. Weiss L. An analysis of the incidence of myocardial metastasis from solid cancers. Br Heart J 1992; 68(5):501–4.

71. Chiles C, Woodard PK, Gutierrez FR, et al. Metastatic involvement of the heart and pericardium: CT and MR imaging. Radiographics 2001;21(2):439–49.

72. Tesolin M, Lapierre C, Oligny L, et al. Cardiac metastases from melanoma. Radiographics 2005;25(1): 249–53.

73. Fujita N, Caputo GR, Higgins CB. Diagnosis and characterization of intracardiac masses by magnetic resonance imaging. Am J Card Imaging 1994;8(1): 69–80.

74. Higgins C. Acquired heart disease. 3rd edition. Philadelphia: Lippincott-Raven; 1997. p. 409–60.

75. Algra PR, Bloem JL, Tissing H, et al. Detection of vertebral metastases: comparison between MR imaging and bone scintigraphy. Radiographics 1991;11(2):219–32.

76. Frank JA, Ling A, Patronas NJ, et al. Detection of malignant bone tumors: MR imaging vs scintigraphy. AJR Am J Roentgenol 1990;155(5): 1043–8.

77. Schmidt GP, Reiser MF, Baur-Melnyk A. Whole-body imaging of bone marrow. Semin Musculoskelet Radiol 2009;13(2):120–33.

78. Lecouvet FE, Malghem J, Michaux L, et al. Skeletal survey in advanced multiple myeloma: radiographic versus MR imaging survey. Br J Haematol 1999; 106(1):35–9.

79. Poitout D, Gaujoux G, Lempidakis M, et al. X-ray computed tomography or MRI in the assessment of bone tumor extension. Chirurgie 1991;117(5–6): 488–90 [in French].

80. Plaza JA, Perez-Montiel D, Mayerson J, et al. Metastases to soft tissue: a review of 118 cases over a 30-year period. Cancer 2008;112(1):193–203.

81. Herring CL Jr, Harrelson JM, Scully SP. Metastatic carcinoma to skeletal muscle. A report of 15 patients. Clin Orthop Relat Res 1998;355:272–81.

82. Stulc JP, Petrelli NJ, Herrera L, et al. Isolated metachronous metastases to soft tissues of the buttock from a colonic adenocarcinoma. Dis Colon Rectum 1985;28(2):117–21.

Recurrence of Melanoma

Sergi Vidal-Sicart, MD, PhD[a,b,c,]*, Domenico Rubello, MD[d],
Francesca Pons, MD, PhD[a,b]

KEYWORDS

- Melanoma • Positron emission tomography (PET)
- Computed tomography (CT) • PET/CT • Recurrence

Although melanoma now accounts for only 4% of all skin cancers, it is responsible for the greatest number of deaths related to skin cancer worldwide. When this finding is compared with figures from 2000 (1 in every 90 people) a startling difference appears: the estimated incidence has now increased to 1 in every 75 individuals.[1] There has been a 3-fold increase in reported cases in middle-aged men and a 5-fold increase in older men over a similar period. The possibility of cure is highest when melanoma is treated in its early stages. The survival rates for patients with cutaneous melanoma are higher in developed countries (81% in Europe) than in developing countries (approximately 40%).[2–5]

As with nearly all malignancies, the possibility of curing melanoma depends on the stage at presentation. It is estimated that 82% to 85% of patients with melanoma present with localized disease, 10% to 13% with regional disease, and 2% to 5% with distant metastatic disease.[6] When melanoma returns after treatment, it is referred to as recurrent. Recurrent melanoma can be local (at or near the site of the original tumor), nodal (stage III), or in another part of the body (stage IV). When melanoma cells spread from the primary tumor, they usually pass through the nearest lymph channel. If this process occurs, there is a risk that they will also appear in other lymph nodes and organs.

PET using [^{18}F]fluorodeoxyglucose (FDG) is a powerful tool in the search for cancer deposits. Staging of patients with melanoma by means of whole-body functional imaging in a single evaluation session using FDG-PET has created much interest over the last decade. FDG-PET has the potential to show tumor metabolic activity before structural changes can be seen by other methods such as computed tomography (CT) imaging. A potential benefit of FDG-PET for patient outcome is the ability to improve the selection of patients for surgery and other treatments. Before the advent of PET, it was difficult to monitor patients for recurrence of cutaneous melanoma, and it has been shown that FDG-PET has a strong role in detection of metastatic disease. FDG-PET can highlight metastases at unusual sites that are easily missed with conventional imaging modalities. It is more sensitive than CT for detection of metastatic lesions in the skin, lymph nodes, and abdomen. Despite the overall superiority of FDG-PET in the detection of melanoma metastases, it has limitations in detection of early-stage disease (stage I–II), small lung nodules, and brain metastases.

RECURRENCE

Although it is relatively easy to predict where melanoma is most likely to spread, it is still not clear why different cancers are more likely to metastasize to specific sites. The following 3 hypotheses have been put forward in an attempt to explain this behavior: the first is that although cancerous cells can colonize indiscriminately at any distant site, they multiply only in those sites that have appropriate cellular growth factors; second, it has been suggested that cancerous cells become glued to specific sites; and third, cancerous cells

[a] Department of Nuclear Medicine, Hospital Clinic, University of Barcelona, Villarroel 170, 08036 Barcelona, Spain
[b] Institut d'Investigacions Biomèdiques August Pi Sunyer (IDIBAPS), Villarroel 170, 08036 Barcelona, Spain
[c] Department of Nuclear Medicine, CRC-MAR, Corporació Sanitària. Passeig Marítim 25, 08003 Barcelona, Spain
[d] Department of Nuclear Medicine, PET/CT Center, Santa Maria della Misericordia Hospital, Viale Tre Martiri 140, 45100 Rovigo, Italy
* Corresponding author. Department of Nuclear Medicine, Hospital Clínic, University of Barcelona, Villarroel 170, 08036 Barcelona, Spain.
E-mail address: svidal@clinic.ub.es

PET Clin 6 (2011) 55–70
doi:10.1016/j.cpet.2010.12.004

may be selectively attracted to specific sites by organ-specific molecules in a process referred to as chemoattraction.[7–9]

The probability that melanoma recurs after appropriate treatment can be characterized as low-risk, intermediate-risk, or high-risk. The low-risk group implies a risk of recurrence of less than 20%, the intermediate-risk group presents a 20% to 50% risk of recurrence, and high risk refers to a greater than 50% risk of recurrence, when there is a high probability that the melanoma has already spread to local or distant sites at the time of treatment.

The risk of recurrence increases with the thickness of the primary tumor (with thicker tumors carrying the greater risk), the presence of ulceration in the primary tumor, and the presence of satellite metastases surrounding the primary tumor.

Types of Recurrence

Local recurrence

A melanoma that develops at or near the site where the primary melanoma was completely removed is called local recurrence and can occur months or years after surgical removal of the primary tumor. Survival rate is generally low. Anatomically, local recurrence is when 1 of the following is found: regrowth of an incompletely excised primary melanoma involving the excision site scar or graft (persistent melanoma) or local metastasis at the primary site.

Local recurrence can be found in association with disseminated disease. Approximately 25% to 30% of patients with American Joint Committee on Cancer (AJCC) stage I to II melanoma have some type of recurrence. In retrospective series with a prolonged follow-up, local recurrence has been reported in up to 10% of patients. New attempts to explain local recurrence define it as a form of lymphatic metastasis that is distinct from regrowth of neoplastic tissue that had been incompletely excised from the site of a previous primary melanoma. It is considered that local recurrence, satellites, and in-transit metastases are likely to be manifestations of lymphatic dissemination.[10]

Regional recurrence

Regional recurrence is recurrence of melanoma seen in the regional lymph node.

There are several factors that predispose patients to a regional recurrence after resection of their primary tumors. Cascinelli and colleagues[11] showed that patients whose nodes tested positive had a higher incidence of recurrence than those with negative nodes. Patients with histologically positive nodes presented in transit disease more often after elective lymph node dissection (27%) than after immediate therapeutic lymph node dissection (4%).

Nodal recurrence is the most common initial site of recurrent disease in patients who have not undergone elective lymph node dissection, whereas visceral metastases are more commonly seen as the first site of failure when elective lymph node dissection has been performed. The factors that predispose to in-transit recurrence are increasing tumor thickness, presence and number of involved nodes, and clinically occult positive lymph nodes.[12]

The information obtained from a sentinel lymph node biopsy plays a key role in regional melanoma staging, but on occasions recurrence has been reported after a histologically negative sentinel node finding (false-negative result). Three potential mechanisms could explain such findings: a technical failure is one in which the true sentinel node was not identified, a pathologic failure is one in which the correct lymph node was harvested but histologic evaluation failed to identify disease, and a biologic failure is one in which residual microscopic satellite or in-transit disease persisted after wide excision of the primary tumor.[13]

Visceral recurrence

Recurrence at a distant visceral site is known as metastatic melanoma (**Fig. 1**). The most common sites for distant recurrences are the lungs, brain, liver, gastrointestinal tract, and bone. Visceral metastases are where relapses are first detected in approximately 25% of all patients with recurrence of melanoma. From 55% to 67% of cases become apparent by 2 years and 65% to 81% by 3 years after definitive treatment of the primary tumor.[12]

The timing and rate of recurrence of melanoma are well documented. Large retrospective studies have shown that 60% to 80% of first recurrences are local and/or nodal. In patients with a lesion thinner than 1.5 mm, the recurrence rate is 2% to 19%. In melanomas that are thicker than 1.5 mm the recurrence rate rises to 47% to 66%. In general, most studies indicate that about 80% of recurrences occur within the first 3 years, but up to 16% of first recurrences have been reported after 5 years or more, and late recurrence (more than 10 years) can also occur.[14–23]

EVALUATION

Whether or not a routine staging examination should be part of the surveillance and follow-up of patients with melanoma is still controversial

A

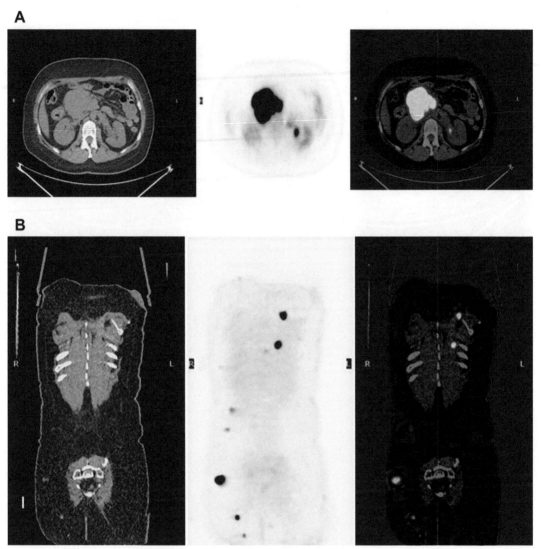

B

Fig. 1. (*A, B, C, D*). Patient with melanoma on the back, which was excised. During follow-up, subcutaneous recurrence was suspected. FDG-PET/CT showed a lot of hypermetabolic lesions on the skin, subcutaneous, abdominal, intestinal and nodal (stage IV). (*Courtesy of* Carlos Trampal, PhD, MD, IAT-CRC Centre d'Imatge Molecular, Barcelona, Spain.)

and several investigators claim that most patients with melanoma can detect their own recurrences.[24,25]

Dalal and colleagues[26] reported that more than half of patients (55%) with early-stage melanoma who underwent wide local excision and a sentinel lymph node biopsy were able to self-detect their recurrences through physical findings or identification of symptoms. In that study, 13% of patients identified in-transit metastases and another 13% nodal disease. A total of 36% local, 61% of in-transit, and 60% of nodal recurrences were self-detected. These results indicate that most recurrences of melanoma are symptomatic and

can be detected by the patient. However, there are valid reasons for a disease evaluation in these patients: one would be to establish a baseline study against which to compare future evaluations in patients at risk of recurrence; it would also serve to detect clinically occult disease, allowing more appropriate treatment decisions to be made.

Because the yield of laboratory tests and imaging studies in patients with stage I to II melanoma for nonsymptomatic metastasis is low,[27] these checks should be performed only when clinically indicated (especially in stage IIb–IIc).[28] In patients classified as stage III with a positive sentinel node, imaging techniques can identify

C

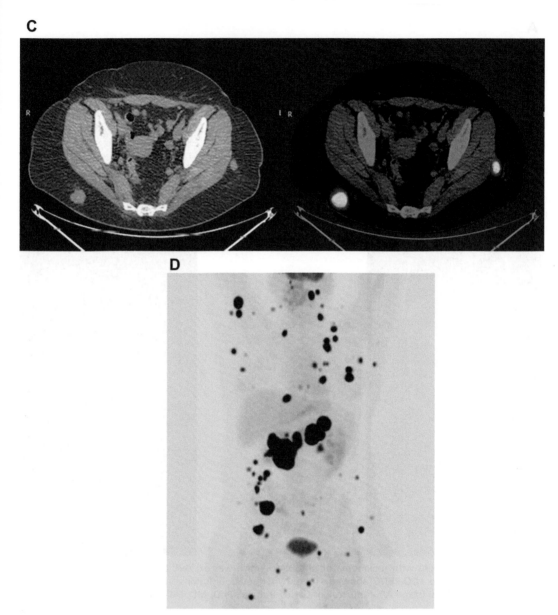

D

Fig. 1. (*continued*)

occult metastases only in 0.5% to 3.7% of cases,[29] but in patients with clinically positive nodes this improves to 4% to 16%. In patients with clinical stage III disease or local recurrence, imaging (especially ultrasound) can give enough information on the lesion for a provisional diagnosis (multiple lesions) and guide a fine-needle biopsy. Ultrasound is useful for early detection of metastatic disease in the regional node field because of its higher sensitivity in discrimination of nodal metastases than palpation.[30] However, despite the superiority of ultrasonography

examination over palpation, benefits can only be seen in 7.2% of patients.[31]

The most accurate method of identifying occult regional lymph node metastases is by sentinel lymph node biopsy. To avoid the risk of a false-negative result using sentinel node, ultrasonography has been widely used to accurately detect lymph node metastases. However, prospective studies have shown that a sentinel lymph node biopsy is superior to ultrasound in the detection of occult regional lymph node metastases.[32] Other studies have compared the sensitivity and specificity of FDG-PET with sentinel node biopsy as the reference standard and found PET inferior to sentinel node, with a sensitivity of only 13% for FDG-PET.[33,34] Another potential use of ultrasonography is to examine the sentinel node to rule out involvement or proceed to lymphadenectomy if fine-needle biopsy shows involvement. It has been reported that between 10% and 16% of patients could be ruled out as candidates for sentinel node biopsy, and these patients can proceed directly to lymph node dissection.[35]

PET scan has been investigated for its potential to detect subclinical metastatic disease. However, most studies have described a low yield and a reduced sensitivity in detecting metastatic melanoma in patients with stage I to II melanoma.[36] Several studies have compared FDG-PET with sentinel lymph node biopsy. Pooling the results, FDG-PET sensitivity was 17% and its specificity 92%, but FDG-PET cannot be used as an alternative to sentinel node biopsy in this setting because of its inability to detect micrometastatic involvement.[31] Crippa and colleagues[37] reported that the sensitivity was 100% for involved nodes larger than 10 mm in size but that this dropped to only 23% in nodes that were smaller than 5 mm.

Although FDG-PET/CT provides improved anatomic information, it has similar limitations to PET in spatial resolution, and the results are similar.[38] In patients with more advanced disease, FDG-PET can characterize doubtful lesions on a CT scan and has the added value of performing a whole-body assessment.[39]

Current National Comprehensive Cancer Network (NCCN) guidelines state that routine imaging techniques (ie, CT, magnetic resonance [MR] imaging, PET) are not recommended for patients with early-stage melanoma and are for use only when signs or symptoms are present. In stage III patients, studies have confirmed that CT or FDG-PET scans are not suitable for screening purposes and ultimately their use is at the clinician's discretion on a case-by-case basis. Nevertheless, in patients with stage IV disease, chest and abdominal/pelvic CT, with or without FDG-PET, and/or head MR imaging, should be considered (especially where there are symptoms of central nervous system involvement). For diagnosis of stage IV melanoma, serum lactate dehydrogenase (LDH) levels should be obtained because of its prognostic role.[28]

FOLLOW-UP

The optimal duration of follow-up remains controversial. Most patients who are going to experience a recurrence of their disease present it in the first 5 years after initial treatment, but late recurrence (after 10 years) has been well documented.[40] In a retrospective study of 2000 patients in stages I to III and more than 10,000 technical examinations, Garbe and colleagues[10] found that 83% of all recurrences were detected during the regular follow-up examinations, with only 17% coming from patients' self-diagnosis. About 50% of all recurrences were detected at an early phase and complete surgical removal was possible. Detection of recurrence at an early phase was associated with a prolonged survival time.

It is important for patients to be aware that melanoma can spread silently (ie, without noticeable symptoms), making follow-up examinations vital. The basic role of follow-up with any patient who has cancer is that early detection of recurrence leads to treatment starting sooner, which could, in turn, have a positive effect on outcome. However, recurrence is not always treatable, and treatment may not guarantee a cure. It is difficult to find a balance between intensity of follow-up and successful outcome in patients with melanoma. Because early detection of recurrence is an important goal of melanoma surveillance, it would be logical to follow these patients at more frequent intervals. The length of time before recurrence is known to vary inversely with the primary tumor thickness. In general, patients who had thinner primary lesions have later recurrence. Early and late recurrence show a similar pattern of spread and prognosis.[41]

Locoregional Disease

It is current practice that all patients with an invasive melanoma who are at risk of recurrence receive a period of follow-up, and in all patients with stage III disease this follow-up is automatically prolonged, often for the rest of their life. There is no risk of recurrence for patients with melanoma in situ.[24] Once a primary cutaneous melanoma has been diagnosed, all future clinical and imaging explorations are aimed at the detection of occult regional systemic disease. A second aim is to identify occult disease stage III or IV not suggested by clinical history or examination, which would result in a change in management. In patients with locoregional recurrence, the aim of routine investigations is to provide more accurate prognostic information and to check for occult stage IV disease, in which a change in therapeutic approach could improve survival.

Following NCCN guidelines, skin examination and surveillance at least once a year for life are recommended for all patients with melanoma. Clinicians should educate patients in a monthly regimen of skin examinations (together with monthly self-examination of the lymph nodes for stage Ia–IV). Laboratory tests and/or imaging are indicated to rule out specific signs and symptoms. For patients with stage IA to IIA melanoma without evidence of disease, a comprehensive history and physical examination, especially in lymph node regional basins and skin, every 3 to 12 months for 5 years is mandatory and annually thereafter if clinically indicated. Patients with stage IIB to IV disease should undergo the same physical examination every 3 to 6 months for 2 years and every 3 to 12 months for the following 3 years, reducing to annually thereafter if clinically indicated. Chest radiography, CT, MR imaging, and/or FDG-PET can be used to screen for recurrent or metastatic disease at the physician's discretion (**Fig. 2**).[28]

In a recent study, Veenstra and colleagues[42] reviewed 886 patients with melanoma treated at the Netherlands Cancer Institute and observed a 15% rate of in-transit metastases in patients with a positive sentinel node and a 14% rate in those patients with palpable node disease.

Depending on the physical examination and symptoms, additional imaging tests may be recommended for all types of stage III disease. These tests may include a CT scan, FDG-PET, or MR imaging. Chest radiograph and blood tests, such as LDH level checks, are optional. Some studies have investigated the role of routine radiograph, thoracic-abdominal CT scans and MR imaging in patients with positive sentinel lymph nodes. The yield of these combined investigations was only 0.5% and 1.9% in 2 studies.[43,44] In 1 of these, 14% of all imaging procedures offered indeterminate results, requiring further investigations, some of which were invasive.

Because more than 50% of patients with macroscopic locoregional cutaneous melanoma go on to present distant recurrences, radiologic explorations are being used routinely despite the lack of evidence from randomized trials to support this use. For these patients, a complete blood analysis, serum LDH level test, and chest radiograph should be obtained for future reference. Although advanced imaging studies (CT, MR imaging, PET) have a low success rate in detecting distant metastases, results are better than in patients with stage I and II disease (**Fig. 3**).[45] CT imaging of the chest and abdomen is commonly performed. Although the yield is low, they function as an important baseline for future studies in this high-risk population. Studies have shown true-positive findings of metastatic disease based on CT in 0% to 26% of cases, with most studies reporting rates less than 10%.[46] Brain MR imaging in this group is controversial. Some clinicians

perform the procedure only in symptomatic patients, to rule out central nervous system involvement, whereas others recommend its use before therapy. Aukema and colleagues[47] reported brain metastases revealed by MR imaging in 7% of 70 patients with stage III melanoma without any other evidence of systemic dissemination. Pfannenberg and colleagues[48] found cerebral metastases in 23.4% of their study population (stage III/IV).

More recently, the use of a PET scan has been under study for patients with stage III disease. Results have generally shown PET scans to be superior to conventional imaging for identifying metastatic disease, except in the brain and lung areas. One of the earliest studies with FDG-PET in stage III patients was made by Gritters and colleagues.[49] These investigators reported a sensitivity of 100% for visceral and abdominal lymph node metastases but a lesser sensitivity for pulmonary metastases, especially if these were less than 1 cm in size.

In patients with positive sentinel node, several investigators have investigated the routine use of FDG-PET to rule out other metastatic involvement. Horn and colleagues[50] reported in 33 patients that PET showed metastases not found with other modalities in 12% of patients. In another study, Constantinidou and colleagues[51] showed false-positive or confusing uptake in 3 of 30 patients with these characteristics. After lymphadenectomy and follow-up, recurrences were depicted in 30% of patients. The results of this study indicate that the routine use of PET as a baseline investigation in asymptomatic patients with positive sentinel node biopsy seems to have only limited value. Fuster and colleagues[52] reported an FDG-PET sensitivity and specificity of 74% and 86%, respectively, for lesion detection in patients with melanoma compared with 58% and 45% using standard imaging. Crippa and colleagues[37] reported a sensitivity, specificity, accuracy, and positive and negative predictive values in detection of lymph node metastases of 95%, 84%, 91%, 92%, and 89%, respectively.

Other studies have shown similar results. Schwimmer and colleagues[53] reported a sensitivity and specificity for recurrence detection of 92% and 90%, respectively. Holder and colleagues[54] obtained a 94.2% sensitivity and 83.3% specificity for FDG-PET and 55.3% and 84.4% for CT, respectively. Mijnhout and colleagues[55] performed a meta-analysis of 6 studies that showed a pooled sensitivity of 79% and a specificity rising to 86%. In their study of 105 patients, Borrego and colleagues[56] reported excellent results in sensitivity (97%), specificity (97.2%), positive predictive

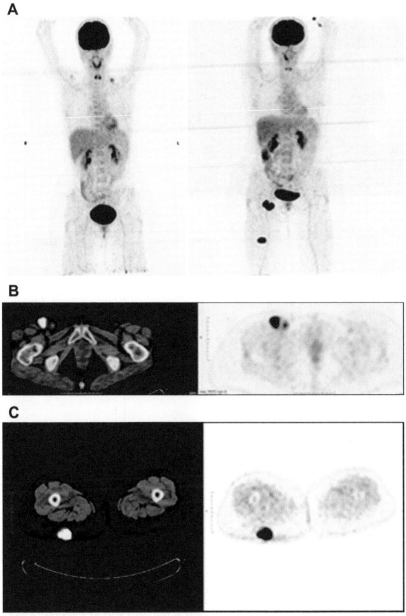

Fig. 2. (*A, B, C*). A patient with a 3-mm Breslow thickness melanoma on the right foot underwent wide local excision with 2-cm margins and sentinel lymph node biopsy. Pathologic analysis did not show metastatic involvement in 2 inguinal sentinel nodes. One year later, FDG-PET/CT scan showed a cutaneous as well as regional recurrence. (*Courtesy of* Renato A. Valdés-Olmos, PhD, MD, Netherlands Cancer Institute-Antoni van Leeuwenhoek Hospital, Amsterdam, The Netherlands.)

value (98.5%), negative predictive value (82%), and accuracy (94.7%). The use of FDG-PET for patients with clinical stage III melanoma has been recommended by Bastiaannet and colleagues,[57] who suggest that when distant metastases are found and surgery is considered, a complementary CT is indicated. On the other hand, when FDG-PET does not detect metastases, an additional CT is not warranted. When PET or PET/CT are not available, CT is a valid alternative, but if metastasectomy is planned, a complementary FDG-PET is preferable to rule out the presence of other metastases.

The role of PET/CT in clinical stage III melanoma is rapidly evolving but, like stand-alone CT or PET, the interpretation of PET/CT results is complicated by false-negative and false-positive results. PET/ CT may be particularly useful in patients with

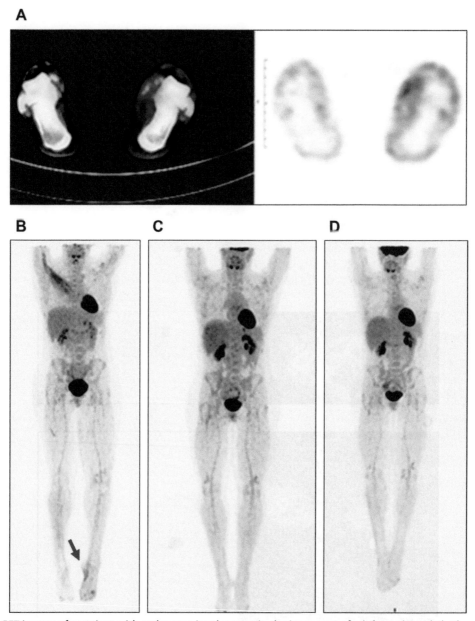

Fig. 3. PET images of a patient with melanoma involvement in the inner part of a left toe (*A* and *B*). The patient underwent surgery in late 2008. Annual imaging follow-up studies did not show recurrence (*C* and *D*). Currently, the patient is disease-free.

advanced locoregional disease, for whom identification of additional regional or systemic involvement could change the planned surgical strategy. Moreover, PET/CT may be used for evaluation of suspicious or misleading findings identified by conventional imaging.[58,59] It is known that PET/CT causes a significant reduction in false-positive results by allowing precise anatomic localization and correlation with morphologic appearances (**Figs. 4** and **5**).

The overall promising results of FDG-PET imaging were confirmed by Reinhardt and colleagues, who assessed 250 patients using PET/CT imaging. The sensitivity, specificity, and accuracy for the N- and M-stage ranged between 95% and 100%. PET alone provided the same high sensitivity as PET/CT for detection of distant lymph node metastases and metastases to all other organs except the lungs. However, the specificity of PET was significantly improved by

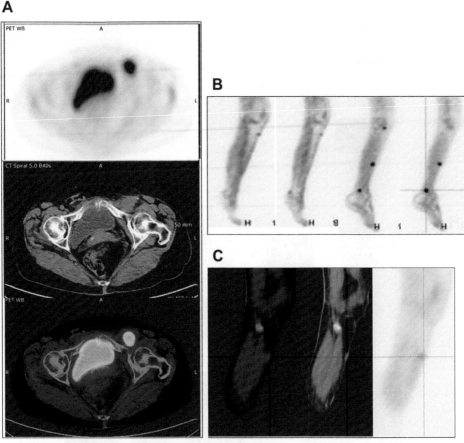

Fig. 4. (*A, B, C*). PET and PET/CT images of a patient with several cutaneous recurrent lesions and inguinal lymph node involvement in a left limb.

imaging fusion with CT, which lowered the incidence of false-positive and false-negative results. The use of PET/CT as a possible first-line modality could be considered for patients with suspected recurrence.[60] Aukema and colleagues[47] showed that FDG-PET/CT had a sensitivity of 87% and a specificity of 98% for staging patients with melanoma with palpable lymph node metastases, and this led to a change in the clinical management in 37% of cases.

False-positive and false-negative findings are potentially disappointing because they can result in incorrect changes of management. Although FDG-PET seems to be an accurate method for recurrent disease or advanced stages in patients with melanoma, if a radical change in the treatment plan is suggested, these FDG-PET findings should be confirmed by biopsy or another test. The number of false-positive cases in PET continues to stand at 10%. The reported causes include inflammation, pneumonia, pseudolymphoma, and endometriosis. Most false-negative findings are

caused by the small volume of metastatic involvement in the lymph nodes, cutis, liver, and lungs. Other options have been described. Strobel and colleagues[61] showed the high relationship between FDG-PET/CT findings and the serum levels of S100B. An increase in S100B serum levels indicates a great likelihood of recurrence and probably a high tumor burden. This finding suggests that a high concentration in S100B levels could be indicative for FDG-PET detection of the disease.

In patients with newly diagnosed stage III disease for whom a potentially morbid treatment is planned that would be abandoned in the presence of metastatic disease, a CT scan of the chest abdomen and pelvis or whole-body PET scan may be performed. No data exist for the role of investigations for those patients with in-transit disease. Hence the recommendations for in-transit disease are the same as for macroscopic stage III disease. For the detection of occult stage III disease, the yields of ultrasound, CT scan, or

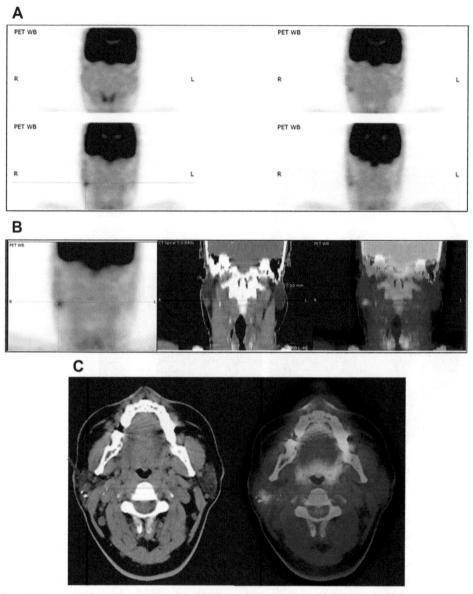

Fig. 5. (*A*, *B*, *C*). Images of a patient with a 2.2-mm nodular melanoma on the right parietal area. Wide excision and sentinel lymph node biopsy were performed. Two preauricular (1 parotideal) sentinel nodes were harvested (negative pathologic report). After 1.5 years a mass was felt in the right parotideal area. A nodal recurrence near the previous surgical field is depicted on the images (*arrow*).

FDG-PET whole-body exploration are inferior to sentinel node biopsy and have been shown to be cost-inefficient.[36,62] It has been suggested that PET should be considered as the first-line imaging procedure for recurrent disease because it has a higher sensitivity and specificity than CT in several series.[63,64] These studies reported sensitivities of PET and CT of 74% to 85% and 58% to 81%, respectively. The specificities for PET and CT were 86% to 97% and 45% to 87%, respectively. PET/CT might have a role in selected

patients from this group because of its better anatomic information and ability to decrease the number of false-positive and false-negative results. Therefore, the use of PET/CT as a possible first-line modality may be suggested in patients with suspected recurrence.

Visceral Recurrences

The body of evidence does not contain any randomized trials to support or exclude the routine use of investigations following the diagnosis of stage IV cutaneous melanoma. Most studies are descriptive or observational. The diagnosis of metastatic melanoma is made from investigations for symptoms or investigations as part of routine follow-up.

Image-guided fine-needle biopsy may be performed to establish the diagnosis of metastatic melanoma when diagnostic doubt remains after imaging studies. Alternatively, clinical observation and serial imaging may be required to confirm the nature of lesions suspected to be metastatic melanoma. Serum LDH forms part of the current AJCC staging system for melanoma and may be measured, once the diagnosis of stage IV melanoma has been established by imaging and/or biopsy, to help in determining the prognosis.

For patients in whom conventional imaging techniques yield misleading results for metastatic melanoma, PET scan should be viewed as a complementary imaging technique. Recently, much attention has been focused on the usefulness of PET scanning in the diagnosis of metastatic melanoma. The sensitivity and specificity of PET scans for the detection of melanoma metastases are reported to be 85% and up to 97%, respectively.[64,65] A recent meta-analysis (n = 753) in this group of patients showed a polled sensitivity of 88% and specificity of 82%, whereas positive predictive value was 92%, negative predictive value 74%, and accuracy was 86%. In detection of the disease, FDG-PET has had good results for regional and mediastinal lymph node metastases, soft-tissue, and bone metastases as well as intraabdominal foci.[31] However, the sensitivity of PET scans decreases to as low as 4% for lesions less than 6 mm in size. Despite

this limitation, PET scans are generally more sensitive than CT scans for the detection of metastatic melanoma at all sites, except for brain and lung.[52,66]

Although the evidence suggests that PET is superior to CT with respect to the number of metastatic sites identified, once the diagnosis of metastatic melanoma has been established by conventional imaging techniques, the supplementary use of PET scans is of little value unless the result would cause a change in management.[67] If surgery is planned for apparently resectable metastatic disease, a sensitive screening test for metastatic disease in other sites, such as PET scanning, might be particularly useful.[68] Several studies have examined the influence of PET scans in addition to conventional imaging in the management of patients with stage IV melanoma who are scheduled for metastasectomy or when the findings are unclear.

The PET results yield a clinical effect in this group of patients under the following conditions:

If they rule out a curative local treatment because of metastatic dissemination or because the lesion is not malignant.

If they lead to a treatment with curative intent.

In this setting, the additional use of a PET scan influenced clinical management by 17% to 49%.[52,57,68–70] Preoperative PET scans are associated with improved outcome after pulmonary metastasectomy by permitting the selection of patients without additional sites that are most likely to benefit from resection. However, when clinical examination and simple imaging have established the presence of inoperable metastatic disease, the addition of PET scanning is of

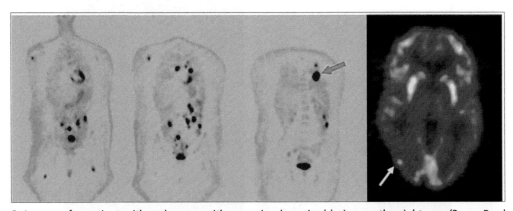

Fig. 6. Images of a patient with melanoma with a previously excised lesion on the right arm (3 mm Breslow). Currently, a solitary recurrence is suspected on the left lung (*green arrow*). Restaging FDG-PET scan also showed multiple nodal lesions in the brain (*yellow arrow*). (*Courtesy of* Carlos Trampal, PhD, MD, IAT-CRC Centre d'Imatge Molecular, Barcelona, Spain.)

questionable value. Serial CT scans are the best method for assessing response to treatment. Although not recommended for routine screening, MR imaging is the most sensitive test for detection of cerebral metastases because the combination of hemorrhage and the presence of melanin combine to give a high-signal intensity on T1-weighted images. However, in symptomatic patients, a brain scan could prove useful to assess the possibility of FDG-avid metastases (Fig. 6).

It has been shown that anatomic and functional imaging techniques are important in this group of patients. Patients with malignant melanoma who have suspected nodal or distant metastatic involvement or a high risk of such spread may undergo an FDG-PET/CT scan for staging purposes. The combined imaging modality may also be used to restage patients with melanoma before surgical metastectomy and to confirm suspected recurrence. FDG-PET/CT results in

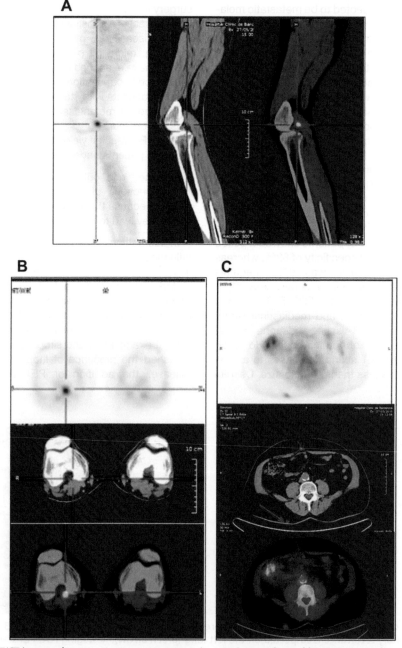

Fig. 7. The PET/CT images show a cutaneous recurrence in a patient with acral lentiginous melanoma on the first toe of the right foot. Popliteal and paralumbar subcutaneous metastases are depicted (*A, B, C,* respectively).

a significant increase in accuracy of 5% to 12%, especially for the increase of sensitivity in the detection of pulmonary metastases in comparison with FDG-PET because of successful detection of small pulmonary nodules by CT component of the device. A diagnostic review of the CT component resulted in a significant improvement in sensitivity (10%) and accuracy (5%).[48,60,61]

There are few reports on soft-tissue metastases, defined as metastases to skeletal muscle and subcutaneous tissue. In patients with melanoma this figure can be as high as 9.8% and it is associated with other distant metastases and is suggestive of poor prognosis (see **Fig. 6**).[71,72] Although MR imaging is not specific for soft-tissue metastasis, it has been advocated as an indispensable tool for diagnosis and treatment planning in patients with soft-tissue malignancy. A recent study showed that FDG-PET/CT has a higher sensitivity than MR imaging in detecting skin and soft-tissue metastasis.[48] This finding supports the increasing role of ^{18}F-FDG-PET/CT in management of patients who have cancer, although it can give false-positive results (actinic keratosis and skin folding). Whole-body PET/CT is typically performed from the skull base to the pelvic floor, because most FDG-avid lesions are expected to be within this field of view (excepting cerebral metastasis). This is most likely why the extremities are not usually included in the field of view unless there is a clinical suspicion for malignancy in the limbs. Nguyen and colleagues[71] found 46% of soft-tissue metastatic lesions in a normal whole-body field of view, suggesting the possibility of underdiagnosis in these patients.

A total whole-body PET/CT scan could be advisable in patients with melanoma to avoid a potential misdiagnosis of soft-tissue lesions. However, this imaging protocol requires additional image acquisition time, resulting in more discomfort for the patient. Löffler and colleagues[72] performed a study to explore the diagnostic benefit of scanning the legs and to evaluate the resulting therapeutic benefits. Recurrent and metastatic disease in the leg was found in 53 of 153 patients, which makes it reasonable to scan the legs in all patients. However, uptake in the legs occurred only with patients who either had a primary lesion in the same area or presented a complete dissemination throughout the body. In patients without previous disease restricted to the legs, a short protocol including torso and proximal thighs can be sufficient, because positive findings seem to be rare in this situation (**Fig. 7**). Now that new advancements in hardware and in software technology in PET/CT are allowing increased scanning without compromising imaging accuracy or time

(ie, time-of-flight technology), it should be possible to evaluate the total body in an adequate time frame.

SUMMARY

When cutaneous melanoma recurrence is suspected, several imaging techniques can be used to confirm or rule out this possibility as well as performing an adequate follow-up of the disease. FDG-PET may play an important role in this setting (recurrent melanoma and stage III/IV), especially in the evaluation of dissemination of the disease when resection of limited metastatic disease is scheduled. However, PET has some limitations, mainly in lungs and brain, for which CT and MR imaging, respectively, are the first-choice techniques. Ultrasonography and FDG-PET can be useful in the assessment of regional node involvement in certain groups of patients, but sentinel node biopsy is currently the gold standard in this setting.

PET/CT in the evaluation and management of patients with advanced locoregional or metastatic disease is evolving quickly. Overall, PET/CT is most useful for identifying all metastatic sites before embarking on a metastasectomy of an apparently isolated lesion or for clarifying the nature of a suspicious lesion identified by CT scan.

REFERENCES

1. Rigel DS, Friedman RJ, Kopf AW. The incidence of malignant melanoma in the United States: issues as we approach the 21st century. J Am Acad Dermatol 1996;34(5 Pt 1):839–47.
2. Jemal A, Siegel R, Ward E, et al. Cancer statistics, 2009. CA Cancer J Clin 2009;59(4):225–49.
3. Cockburn M, Swetter SM, Peng D, et al. Melanoma underreporting: why does it happen, how big is the problem, and how do we fix it? J Am Acad Dermatol 2008;59(6):1081–5.
4. Parkin DM, Bray F, Ferlay J, et al. Global cancer statistics, 2002. CA Cancer J Clin 2005;55(2):74–108.
5. Geller AC, Miller DR, Annas GD, et al. Melanoma incidence and mortality among US whites, 1969–1999. JAMA 2002;288(14):1719–20.
6. Balch CM, Gershenwald JE, Soong SJ, et al. Final version 2009 AJCC melanoma staging and classification. J Clin Oncol 2009;27(36):6199–207.
7. Meier F, Will S, Ellwanger U, et al. Metastatic pathways and time courses in the orderly progression of cutaneous melanoma. Br J Dermatol 2002;147(1):62–70.
8. Nathanson SD. Insights into the mechanisms of lymph node metastasis. Cancer 2003;98(2):413–23.
9. Payne AS, Cornelius LA. The role of chemokines in melanoma tumor growth and metastasis. J Invest Dermatol 2002;118(6):915–22.

10. Gershenwald JE, Balch CM, Soong SJ, et al. Prognostic factors and natural history. In: Balch CM, Houghton AN, Sober AJ, et al, editors. Cutaneous melanoma. 4th edition. St Louis (MO): Quality Medical Publishing; 2003. p. 25–54.

11. Cascinelli N, Morabito A, Santinami M, et al. Immediate or delayed dissection of regional nodes in patients with melanoma of the trunk: a randomised trial. Lancet 1998;351(9105):793–6.

12. Reintgen DS, Cox C, Slingluff CL Jr, et al. Recurrent malignant melanoma: the identification of prognostic factors to predict survival. Ann Plast Surg 1992; 28(1):45–9.

13. Vidal-Sicart S, Pons F, Puig S, et al. Identification of the continel lymph node in patients with malignant melanoma: what are the reasons for mistakes? Eur J Nucl Med 2003;30(3):362–6.

14. Mooney MM, Kulas M, McKinley B, et al. Impact on survival by method of recurrence detection in stage I and II cutaneous melanoma. Ann Surg Oncol 1998; 5(1):54–63.

15. Kelly JW, Blois MS, Sagebiel RW. Frequency and duration of patient follow-up after treatment of a primary malignant melanoma. J Am Acad Dermatol 1985;13(5 Pt 1):756–60.

16. McCarthy WH, Shaw HM, Thompson JF, et al. Time and frequency of recurrence of cutaneous stage I malignant melanoma with guidelines for follow up. Surg Gynecol Obstet 1988;166(6):497–502.

17. Baughan CA, Hall VL, Leppard BJ, et al. Follow up in stage 1 cutaneous malignant melanoma: an audit. Clin Oncol 1993;5(3):174–80.

18. Garbe C, Paul A, Kohler-Spath H, et al. Prospective evaluation of a follow-up schedule in cutaneous melanoma patients: recommendations for an effective follow-up strategy. J Clin Oncol 2003;21(19):520–9.

19. Martini L, Brandini P, Chiarugi C, et al. First recurrence analysis of 840 cutaneous melanomas: a proposal for a follow up schedule. Tumori 1994; 80(2):188–91.

20. Fusi S, Ariyan S, Sternlicht A. Data on first recurrence after treatment for malignant melanoma in a large patient population. Plast Reconstr Surg 1993;91(1):94–8.

21. Tahery DP, Moy RL. Lack of predictive factors in late recurrence of stage 1 melanoma. Int J Dermatol 1992;31(9):629–31.

22. McCarthy WH, Shaw HM, McCarthy SW, et al. Cutaneous melanomas that defy conventional prognostic indicators. Semin Oncol 1996;23(6):709–13.

23. Borgstein PJ, Meijer S, van Diest PJ. Are locoregional cutaneous metastases in melanoma predictable? Ann Surg Oncol 1999;6(3):315–21.

24. Dicker TJ, Kavanagh GM, Herd RM, et al. A rational approach to melanoma follow-up in patients with primary cutaneous melanoma. Scottish Melanoma Group. Br J Dermatol 1999;140(2):249–54.

25. Weiss M, Loprinzi CL, Creagan ET, et al. Utility of follow-up test for detecting recurrent disease in patients with malignant melanomas. JAMA 1995; 274(21):1703–5.

26. Dalal KM, Zhou Q, Panageas KS, et al. Methods of detection of first recurrence in patients with stage I/II primary cutaneous melanoma after sentinel lymph node biopsy. Ann Surg Oncol 2008;15(8): 2206–14.

27. Wang TS, Johnson TM, Cascade PN, et al. Evaluation of staging chest radiographs and serum lactate dehydrogenase for localized melanoma. J Am Acad Dermatol 2004;51(3):399–405.

28. National Cancer Comprehensive Network. Clinical practice guidelines in oncology (v.2. 2010). Melanoma. Available at: http://www.nccn.org/professionals/physician.gls/PDF/melanoma.pdf. Accessed June, 2010.

29. Gold JS, Jacques DP, Busam KJ, et al. Yield and predictors of radiologic studies for identifying distant metastases in melanoma patients with a positive sentinel lymph node biopsy. Ann Surg Oncol 2007;14(7):2133–40.

30. Bafounta ML, Beauchet A, Chagnon S, et al. Ultrasonography or palpation for the detection of melanoma nodal invasion: a meta-analysis. Lancet Oncol 2004; 5(11):673–80.

31. Ho Shon IA, Chung DK, Saw RP, et al. Imaging in cutaneous melanoma. Nucl Med Commun 2008; 29(10):847–76.

32. Starrit EC, Uren RF, Scoyler RA, et al. Ultrasound examination of sentinel nodes in the initial assessment of patients with primary cutaneous melanoma. Ann Surg Oncol 2005;12(1):18–23.

33. Havenga K, Cobben DC, Oyen WJ, et al. Fluorodeoxyglucose-positron emission tomography and sentinel lymph node biopsy in staging primary cutaneous melanoma. Eur J Surg Oncol 2003;29(8):662–4.

34. Fink AM, Holle-Robatsch S, Herzog N, et al. Positron emission tomography is not useful in detecting metastasis in the sentinel lymph node in patients with primary malignant melanoma stage I and II. Melanoma Res 2004;14(2):141–5.

35. Voit C, Kron M, Schafer G, et al. Ultrasound-guided fine needle aspiration cytology prior to sentinel lymph node biopsy in melanoma patients. Ann Surg Oncol 2006;13(12):1682–9.

36. Wagner JD, Schauwecker D, Davidson D, et al. Inefficacy of F-18 fluorodeoxy-D-glucose-positron emission tomography scans for initial evaluation in early-stage cutaneous melanoma. Cancer 2005;104(3):570–9.

37. Crippa F, Leutner M, Belli F, et al. Which kinds of lymph node metastases can FDG PET detect? A clinical study in melanoma. J Nucl Med 2000;41(9):1491–4.

38. Kell MR, Ridge JA, Joseph N, et al. PET-CT imaging in patients undergoing sentinel node biopsy for melanoma. Eur J Surg Oncol 2007;33(7):911–3.

39. Brady MS, Akhurst T, Spanknebel K, et al. Utility of preoperative 18F fluorodeoxyglucose-positron emission tomography scanning in high-risk melanoma patients. Ann Surg Oncol 2006;13(4):525–32.

40. Crowley NJ, Seigler HF. Late recurrence of malignant melanoma. Analysis of 168 patients. Ann Surg 1990;212(2):173–7.

41. Crowley NJ, Seigler HF. Relationship between disease-free interval and survival in patients with recurrent melanoma. Arch Surg 1992;127(11): 1303–8.

42. Veenstra HJ, van der Ploeg IMC, Wouters MW, et al. Reevaluation of the locoregional recurrence rate in melanoma patients with a positive sentinel node compared to patients with palpable nodal involvement. Ann Surg Oncol 2010;17(2):521–6.

43. Aloia TA, Gershenwald JE, Andtbacka RH, et al. Utility of computed tomography and magnetic resonance imaging staging before completion lymphadenectomy in patients with sentinel lymph node-positive melanoma. J Clin Oncol 2006; 24(18):2858–65.

44. Miranda EP, Gertner M, Wall J, et al. Routine imaging of asymptomatic melanoma patients with metastasis to sentinel lymph nodes rarely identifies systemic disease. Arch Surg 2004;139(8):831–6.

45. Mohr P, Eggermont AM, Hauschild A, et al. Staging of cutaneous melanoma. Ann Oncol 2009;20(Suppl 6): vi14–21.

46. Kuvshinoff BW, Kurtz C, Coit DG. Computed tomography in the evaluation of patients with stage III melanoma. Ann Surg Oncol 1997;4(3):252–8.

47. Aukema TS, Valdes-Olmos RA, Wouters MW, et al. Utility of preoperative 18F-FDG PET/CT and brain MRI in melanoma patients with palpable lymph node metastasis. Ann Surg Oncol 2010;17(10):2773–8.

48. Pfannenberg C, Aschoff P, Schanz S, et al. Prospective comparison of 18F-fluorodeoxyglucose positron emission tomography/computed tomography and whole body magnetic resonance imaging in staging of advanced malignant melanoma. Eur J Cancer 2007;43(3):557–64.

49. Gritters LS, Francis IR, Zasadny KR, et al. Initial assessment of positron emission tomography using 2-fluorine-18-fluoro-2-deoxy-D-glucose in the imaging of malignant melanoma. J Nucl Med 1993; 34(9):1420–7.

50. Horn J, Lock-Andersen J, Sjostrand H, et al. Routine use of FDG-PET scans in melanoma patients with positive sentinel node biopsy. Eur J Nucl Med Mol Imaging 2006;33(8):887–92.

51. Constantinidou A, Hofman M, O'Doherty M, et al. Routine positron emission tomography and positron emission tomography/computed tomography in melanoma staging with positive sentinel node biopsy is of limited benefit. Melanoma Res 2008; 18(1):56–60.

52. Fuster D, Chiang S, Johnson G, et al. Is 18F-FDG PET more accurate than standard diagnostic procedures in the detection of suspected recurrent melanoma? J Nucl Med 2004;45(8):1323–7.

53. Schwimmor J, Essner R, Patel A, et al. A review of the literature for whole-body FDG PET in the management of patients with melanoma. Q J Nucl Med 2000;44(2):153–67.

54. Holder WD, White RL, Zuger JH, et al. Effectiveness of positron emission tomography for the detection of melanoma metastases. Ann Surg 1998;227(5):764–71.

55. Mijnhout GS, Hoekstra OS, van Tulder MW, et al. Systematic review of the diagnostic accuracy of 18F-fluorodeoxyglucose positron emission tomography in melanoma patients. Cancer 2001;91(8): 1530–41.

56. Borrego I, Vazquez R, Lopez J, et al. Evaluation of efficacy and clinical impact of FDG-PET on patients with suspicion of recurrent cutaneous melanoma. Rev Esp Med Nucl 2006;25(5):301–11.

57. Bastiaannet E, Wobbes T, Hoekstra OS, et al. Prospective comparison of 18F fluorodeoxyglucose positron emission tomography and computed tomography in patients with melanoma with palpable lymph node metastases: diagnostic accuracy and impact on treatment. J Clin Oncol 2009; 27(28):4774–80.

58. Belhocine TZ, Scott AM, Even-Sapir E, et al. Role of nuclear medicine in the management of cutaneous malignant melanoma. J Nucl Med 2006; 47(6):957–67.

59. Garbe C, Eigentler TK. Diagnosis and treatment of cutaneous melanoma. State of the art 2006. Melanoma Res 2007;17(2):117–27.

60. Reinhardt MJ, Joe AY, Jaeger U, et al. Diagnostic performance of whole body dual modality 18F FDG PET/CT imaging for N- and M-staging of malignant melanoma: experience with 250 consecutive patients. J Clin Oncol 2006;24(7):1178–87.

61. Strobel K, Dummer R, Husarik DB, et al. High-risk melanoma: accuracy of FDG PET/CT with added CT morphologic information for detection of metastases. Radiology 2007;244(2):566–74.

62. Hofmann U, Szedlak M, Rittgen W, et al. Primary staging and follow-up in melanoma patients–monocenter evaluation and methods, costs and patient survival. Br J Cancer 2002;87(2):151–7.

63. Stas M, Stroobants S, Dupont P, et al. 18F-FDG PET scan in the staging of recurrent melanoma: Additional value and therapeutic impact. Melanoma Res 2002;12(5):479–90.

64. Swetter SM, Carroll LA, Johnson DL, et al. Positron emission tomography is superior to computed tomography for metastatic detection in melanoma patients. Ann Surg Oncol 2002;9(7):646–53.

65. Schauwecker DS, Siddiqui AR, Wagner JD, et al. Melanoma patients evaluated by four different

positron emission tomography reconstruction techniques. Nucl Med Commun 2003;24(3):281–9.

66. Dietlin M, Krug B, Groth W, et al. Positron emission tomography using 18F-fluorodeoxyglucose in advanced stages of malignant melanoma: a comparison of ultrasonographic and radiological methods of diagnosis. Nucl Med Commun 1999;20(3):255–61.

67. Krug B, Dietlein M, Groth W, et al. Fluor-18-florodeoxuglucose positron emission tomography (FDG-PET) in malignant melanoma. Diagnostic comparison with conventional imaging methods. Acta Radiol 2000;41(5):446–52.

68. Eigtved A, Andersson AP, Dahlstrom K, et al. Use of fluorine-18 fluorodeoxyglucose positron emission tomography in the detection of silent metastases from malignant melanoma. Eur J Nucl Med 2000; 27(1):70–5.

69. Gulec SA, Faries MB, Lee CC, et al. The role of fluorine-18 deoxyglucose positron emission tomography in the management of patients with metastatic melanoma: impact on surgical decision making. Clin Nucl Med 2003;28(12):961–5.

70. Harris MT, Berlangieri SU, Cebon JS, et al. Impact of 2-deoxy-s(18F)fluoro-D-glucose positron emission tomography on the management of patients with advanced melanoma. Mol Imag Biol 2005;23(4):1–5.

71. Nguyen NC, Chaar B, Osman M. Prevalence and patterns of soft tissue metastasis: detection with true whole-body F-18 PET/CT. BMC Med Imaging 2007;7:8–15.

72. Löffler M, Weckesser M, Franzius CH, et al. Malignant melanoma and 18F-FDG-PET: should the whole body scan include the legs? Nuklearmedizin 2003; 42(4):167–72.

Preclinical Studies with Small Animal PET

Cristina Nanni, MD*, Stefano Fanti, MD

KEYWORDS

- Small animals • Positron emission tomography
- Preclinical studies

Cutaneous malignant melanoma is one of the most lethal and almost incurable cancers, characterized by increasing incidence, especially in Europe and the United States.[1,2] Five-year survival is only 15% when widespread metastatic deposits are present but increases to 99% if the disease is detected before it has spread.[3] Although research is active in this field, effective therapies are not available yet and early diagnosis and accurate staging are the most important factors related to a prolonged survival.[4,5] Consequently, it is clear how relevant molecular imaging compounds could be for the evaluation of patients with melanoma.

Currently, [18F]fluorodeoxyglucose (FDG)-PET and PET/computed tomography (CT) are widely used in staging melanoma, which is recognized to be a highly metabolic disease. The sensitivity, specificity, and accuracy of [18F]FDG-PET for detecting recurrent melanoma in human patients range from 70% to 100%.[3] However, because of the inability in detecting micrometastasis, the sensitivity for the identification of sentinel lymph node goes down to 17.3% (0%–40%), which is insufficient for clinical purposes. Also other small lesions could be missed and the brain (a site of secondary lesions) is almost unexplorable because of the physiologic, highly increased, background activity.[3]

Moreover, because the mechanism of uptake and cellular retention of [18F]FDG involves increased glucose metabolism, which may also be seen in many other tumor types and in inflammatory conditions, this tracer lacks specificity for melanoma.[6,7]

Therefore, there is a need to develop imaging agents with higher sensitivity and specificity for small lesions and for the detection of sentinel lymph node metastases as well as molecular probes that can visualize the expression and activity of other molecular targets and biologic processes in melanoma.

The development of new PET probes selective for melanoma cells is confined to the preclinical field, and several micro-PET studies have been published, with satisfying results.

The most important metabolic processes that have been explored are the targeting of melanocortin-1 receptor (overexpressed on melanoma cells surface), the synthesis of melanin and, of course, the intracellular glucose consumption.

SMALL ANIMAL PET

The most sophisticated imaging techniques related to the molecular imaging field belong to nuclear medicine, and are based on the use of radioactive isotopes to label several molecular probes.

According to the physical characteristics of the isotope, it is possible to distinguish the PET imaging that is based on positron emitter isotopes, from the single photon emission computed tomography (SPECT) imaging that is based on γ emitter isotopes.

PET imaging has some advantages over SPECT. The most important is that it is possible to label physiologic molecules (eg, glucose or amino acids or receptor ligands) with positron emitter isotopes without changing the molecule shape (especially if the isotope is ^{11}C, which is normally present in all the organic molecules) to observe its physiologic kinetic in vivo, or making some specific changes in the molecule shape to

UO Medicina Nucleare, Azienda Ospedaliero Universitaria di Bologna Policlinico S.Orsola-Malpighi, Via Massarenti n.9, 40138 Bologna, Italy
* Corresponding author.
E-mail address: cristina.nanni@aosp.bo.it

PET Clin 6 (2011) 71–77
doi:10.1016/j.cpet.2010.12.003

cause a specific block in its metabolism (eg, [^{18}F] FDG).

In recent years,[8,9] a great advance in the technological field allowed small PET tomographs with small gantries to be built, significantly improving the spatial resolution, which is now less than 2 mm. This characteristic is an advantage because the anatomic structures of a mouse are tiny, and a standard spatial resolution of 5 mm (characteristic of clinical scanners) is sometimes not enough.

Another advantage of PET imaging applied to small animal analysis is the sensitivity of this technique, which is able to detect nanograms of tracer in vivo, allowing observation of even molecular events at low concentrations.

Small animal PET (SA-PET) can be used in several preclinical research fields, the most important of which are oncology, cardiology, and neurology.[10,11]

For oncology, SA-PET allows noninvasive measurement of a range of tumor-relevant parameters at both the cellular and the molecular level (eg, the tumor response to an experimental therapeutic intervention,[12] the tumor kinetic of growth, the tumor receptor profile, the tumor vascularization or hypoxia, the tumor proliferative index).[13] The most widely used PET imaging probe is ^{18}F-labeled deoxyglucose, which achieves tumor-specific accumulation on the basis that tumor cells have a higher rate of glucose uptake and metabolism (glycolysis) than normal tissues. FDG is used in oncology to predict cancer cell engraftment[14] and to measure the response to therapy.

Many other PET probes are under development to obtain more tumor specificity via a variety of tumor-specific mechanisms, because virtually all the biologic molecules can be labeled.

The main disadvantage of SA-PET imaging is the high cost of the scanners and the need to work close to a cyclotron-based radiopharmacy, which must be equipped to synthesize novel and experimental probes. Furthermore, the PET diagnostic may present some inconvenience in detecting nonfocal spread of cancer cells, and animal models of cancer must be properly designed for imaging purposes (eg, peritoneal diffusion is frequently missed, whereas subcutaneous implants of cancer cells are more detectable) (**Figs. 1** and **2**).

α-MELANOCYTE-STIMULATING HORMONE PEPTIDE ANALOGUE

The α-melanocyte-stimulating hormone (α-MSH) receptor (melanocortin type 1 receptor [MC1R]) plays an important role in the proliferation and differentiation of melanocytes as well as in the development and growth of melanoma cells. It is considered a genetic link to skin cancer.[15] The MC1R is overexpressed in most murine and human melanoma metastases,[16,17] thus making it a promising molecular target for imaging and therapy for melanomas.

Various α-MSH peptides radiolabeled with ^{18}F,[18] ^{99m}Tc,[19,20] ^{111}In,[21–26] ^{125}I,[27] ^{67}Ga,[28] ^{86}Y,[29] and ^{64}Cu[29–33] that can recognize the MC1R in vitro or in vivo have been prepared and evaluated for melanoma detection. Moreover, an α-MSH peptide, ReCCMSH (Arg11), radiolabeled with a therapeutic radionuclide (either ^{188}Re or ^{212}Pb) has shown promising therapeutic efficacy in mice bearing either B16F1 murine or TXM13 human xenografted melanoma.[23,24] These results highlight the potential of using α-MSH analogues tagged with radionuclides for metastatic melanoma imaging or peptide receptor-targeted radionuclide therapy. For different human and murine melanoma cell lines, the MC1R expression ranges from several hundred to around 10,000 receptors per cell,[16] which is enough for detecting selective imaging probes.

Wei and colleagues[34] tested in vivo the melanoma-targeting peptide (Arg11)CCMSH, which was cyclized by reincorporation to yield CHX-A″-Re(Arg11)CCMSH. They labeled CHX-A″-Re(Arg11)CCMSH with ^{111}In, ^{86}Y, and ^{68}Ga, and the radiolabeled peptides were examined in B16/F1 melanoma-bearing mice for their pharmacokinetic as well as their tumor-targeting properties using SA-SPECT and -PET. The specificity of the binding was shown by injecting a nonradiolabeled peptide before the tracer injection, to cause a cold and specific block of the receptor.

These investigators found radiolabeling efficiencies of the ^{111}In-, ^{86}Y-, and ^{68}Ga-labeled CHX-A″-Re(Arg11)CCMSH peptides were >95%, resulting in specific activities of 4.44, 3.7, and 1.85 MBq/μg, respectively. Tumor uptake of the ^{111}In-, ^{86}Y-, and ^{68}Ga-labeled peptides was rapid and the amount of tracer within the tumor was enough for imaging 2 hours after injection. Disappearance of radioactivity from the normal organs and tissues was rapid as well, with the exception of the kidneys. Melanoma tumors were imaged with all 3 radiolabeled peptides 2 hours after injection. MC1R-specific uptake was confirmed by competitive receptor-blocking studies.

The same group published another paper more focused on the performances of ^{68}Ga-labeled DOTA-rhenium-cyclized α-MSH analogue[35] for imaging melanoma in small animal models. Biodistribution studies showed moderate receptor-mediated tumor uptake, fast nontarget organ clearance, and high tumor/nontarget tissue ratios.

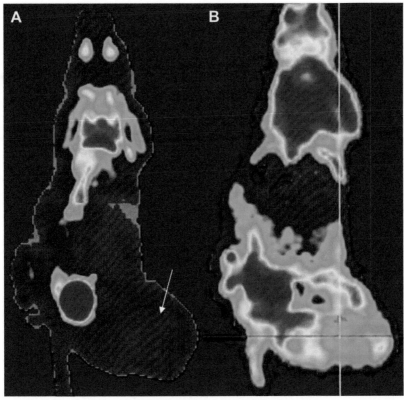

Fig. 1. Xenograft mouse model of melanoma evaluated with 2 tracers by SA-PET. Those animals were inoculated with an M20 cell line in the right inferior limb. (*A*) FDG-SA-PET maximum intensity projection image showing a moderate increased uptake in the neoplastic mass (*arrow*). (*B*) FDG-SA-PET coronal image showing a moderate increased uptake in the neoplastic mass (*cross*) with central necrosis (*cold central area*).

Preadministration of D-lysine significantly reduced kidney uptake without affecting the uptake of the agent in the tumor. SA-PET images showed that the tumor could be clearly visualized at all time points examined (0.5–2 hours) with the standardized uptake value analysis following a similar trend to the biodistribution data.

[68]Ga was also selected as a labeling isotope to label a DOTA-α-melanocyte-stimulating hormone analogue by Froidevaux and coworkers.[28] A short linear α-MSH analogue, [Nle4,Asp5,D-Phe7]-α-MSH4–11 (NAPamide), was designed and conjugated to the metal chelator DOTA (1,4,7,10-tetraazacyclododecane-1,4,7,10-tetraacetic acid) to enable radiometal incorporation. DOTA-NAPamide was conjugated with ^{111}In, ^{67}Ga, and ^{68}Ga and exhibited an almost 7-fold-higher MC1R binding potency compared with DOTA-MSHoct, a previous compound tested by the same group. In melanoma-bearing mice, both ^{111}In-DOTA-NAPamide and ^{67}Ga-DOTA-NAPamide behaved more favorably than ^{111}In-DOTA-MSHoct. Both radiopeptides showed higher tumor

and lower kidney uptake, leading to tumor/kidney ratios of the 4- to 48-hour area under the curve that were 4.6 times (^{111}In) and 7.5 times (^{67}Ga) greater than that obtained with ^{111}In-DOTA-MSHoct.

Skin primary melanoma as well as lung and liver melanoma metastases could be easily visualized on tissue section autoradiographs after systemic injection of ^{67}Ga-DOTA-NAPamide. The melanoma selectivity of DOTA-NAPamide was confirmed by PET imaging studies using ^{68}Ga-DOTA-NAPamide. Tumor uptake was found to be highest when the smallest amount of peptide was administered.

Another paper by Cheng and coworkers[36] tested an ^{18}F-labeled compound, another α-MSH analogue, Ac-Nle-Asp-His-DPhe-Arg-Trp-Gly-Lys-NH2 (NAPamide) that was radiolabeled with N-succinimidyl-4-[^{18}F]fluorobenzoate ([^{18}F]SFB). The resulting radiopeptide was evaluated as a potential molecular probe for SA-PET of melanoma and MC1R expression in melanoma-xenografted mouse models. The investigators found a good binding

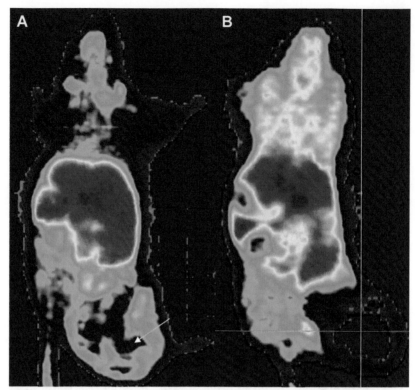

Fig. 2. (A) [^{11}C]Methionine SA-PET maximum intensity projection image showing a moderate-to-high increased uptake in the neoplastic mass (*arrow*). (B) [^{11}C]Methionine SA-PET maximum intensity projection image showing a moderate-to-high increased uptake in the neoplastic mass (*cross*) with central necrosis (*cold central area*).

activity in vitro and a favorable biodistribution in vivo that was completely inhibited by a selective blocker of the receptor.

The same group from Stanford University[37] subsequently tested other tracers targeted to α-MSH receptor. Two ^{18}F-labeled metallopeptides (2 isomers of the same molecule, Ac-D-Lys-ReCCMSH(Arg11) labeled with N-succinimidyl-4-[^{18}F]fluorobenzoate) were proved to have a good affinity to the receptor and good image quality on animal models of melanoma evaluated with SA-PET, although the isoform-1 turned out to provide higher uptake within the tumor.

MELANIN-TARGETED PET TRACERS

In recent years, several other radiolabeled imaging probes have been evaluated for melanoma imaging, including methylene blue dye, monoclonal antibodies direct against melanoma-associated antigens, iodoamphetamine, α-melanocyte-stimulating hormone analogue, and benzamide (BZA)-based compounds. Iodinated BZA analogues have been among the most promising of the newer melanoma radiotracers for both diagnosis and therapeutic applications.

Clinical trials have shown the usefulness of [^{123}I]N-(2-diethylaminoethyl)-4-iodobenzamide ([^{123}I]BZA), [^{123}I]N-(diethylaminoethyl)-2-iodobenzamide ([^{123}I]BZA2), and [^{123}I]iodobenzamide to image cutaneous and ocular melanoma deposits with high specificity and sensitivity.[38–49]

The group from Peter Mac Cancer Center in Melbourne recently evaluated a series of fluoronicotinamide compounds designed specifically for labeling with ^{18}F for melanoma imaging with PET, among which the most promising was MEL050. This compound had excellent tumor uptake, radiochemical stability, and pharmacokinetic properties, with predominant renal excretion.[50] These investigators found that in pigmented B16-F0 grafts, ^{18}F-MEL050 PET yielded a tumor/background ratio of approximately 20:1 at 1 hour and greater than 50:1 at 2 and 3 hours. In the B16-F0 melanoma allograft model, tumor/background ratio was more than 9-fold higher for ^{18}F-MEL050 than for [^{18}F]FDG (50.9 ± 6.9 vs 5.8 ± 0.5). No uptake was observed in the amelanotic melanoma xenografts.

Intense uptake of ^{18}F-MEL050 was evident in metastatic lesions in the lungs of B16-BL6 tumor-bearing mice on PET at 2 hours after tracer injection, with high concordance between ^{18}F-MEL050 accumulation on PET/CT and tumor burden determined at necroscopy.[51]

Similar results were obtained by Ren and colleagues,[52] who tested another BZA analogue labeled with [18]F: N-[2-(diethylamino)-ethyl]-4-[^{18}F] fluorobenzamide ([^{18}F]FBZA). As previously described, this compound showed a high affinity for melanoma cells too, and a high in vivo tumor uptake in SA-PET studies, with a low uptake in mouse models of amelanotic melanoma.

FDG

Because FDG is already widely used for the clinical imaging of patients with melanoma, its use is not diffuse in preclinical imaging research. FDG-PET/CT accuracy and limitations are well known for the evaluation of melanoma extension, despite its overall good accuracy. FDG-PET/CT is not feasible for the localization of flat skin lesions because their depth does not reach the resolution of PET imaging. Lymph node micrometastasis is not detectable and this is an important drawback for the disease staging accuracy. Furthermore, drainage lymph nodes could turn falsely positive in case of inflammation, which is a relatively frequent event because limb melanoma diffuses to inguinal and axillary nodes, which are a common site of benign inflammation.

To better evaluate FDG-PET performance in melanoma and to find an animal model that is feasible for micro-PET imaging, Boisgard and coworkers[53] evaluated a series of 5 melanoblastoma-bearing Libechov minipigs by conducting serial whole-body 2-deoxy-2-[^{18}F] FDG-PET scans. To explore different clinical stages of the tumoral lesions, each animal was scanned 2 to 4 times, at intervals of 30 to 155 days. These investigators performed histology on biopsies taken between or after the scans and the histologic grading of the tumors was compared with the FDG uptake. The overall sensitivity of FDG-PET for the detection of cutaneous melanoma was 75%, and 62.5% of involved lymph nodes were positive. As expected, these investigators found a better sensitivity for tumors with vertical growth than for flat lesions. FDG-PET was not able to detect tumors with epidermal involvement only, nor did it detect small metastatic foci, under the PET resolution limit. Overall, the investigators concluded that, despite some limitations, FDG-PET was effective in the staging of cutaneous melanoma and the follow-up of tumoral extension and regression in their animal model, and that this behavior correlates well with those described in human melanoma. This finding makes this animal model feasible to test new drugs, the effect of which could be evaluated by SA-PET imaging.

SUMMARY

Many new PET probes are under evaluation for the functional imaging of patients with melanoma. Those tracers are targeted to α-MSH receptors and to the intracellular biosynthesis of melanin. Their chemical synthesis and labeling are well-established processes, and so far promising results have been obtained by imaging small animal models of melanoma.

However, no comparison studies are available, and therefore it is impossible to derive which of those tracers leads to the most accurate PET imaging. Furthermore, much work remains to be done before those compounds are available for the routine PET imaging of patients with melanoma.

REFERENCES

1. Jemal A, Murray T, Ward E, et al. Cancer statistics, 2005. CA Cancer J Clin 2005;55:10–30.
2. Thompson JF, Scolyer RA, Kefford RF. Cutaneous melanoma. Lancet 2005;365:687–701.
3. Balch CM, Soong SJ, Atkins MB, et al. An evidence-based staging system for cutaneous melanoma. CA Cancer J Clin 2004;54:131–49.
4. Belhocine TZ, Scott AM, Even-Sapir E, et al. Role of nuclear medicine in the management of cutaneous malignant melanoma. J Nucl Med 2006;27: 957–67.
5. Rohren EM, Turkington TG, Coleman RE. Clinical applications of PET in oncology. Radiology 2004; 231:305–32.
6. Mittra E, Quon A. Positron emission tomography/computed tomography: the current technology and applications. Radiol Clin North Am 2009;47: 147–60.
7. Nabi HA, Zubeldia JM. Clinical applications of 18F-FDG in oncology. J Nucl Med Technol 2002;30:3–9.
8. Sossi V, Ruth TJ. Micropet imaging: in vivo biochemistry in small animals. J Neural Transm 2005;112: 319–30.
9. Weber S, Bauer A. Small animal PET: aspects of performance assessment. Eur J Nucl Med Mol Imaging 2004;31(11):1545–55.
10. Lyons Scott K. Advances in imaging mouse tumour models in vivo. J Pathol 2005;205:194–205.
11. Myers R, Hume S. Small animal PET. Eur Neuropsychopharmacol 2002;12:1545–55.
12. Zhang Y, Saylor M, Wen, et al. Longitudinally quantitative 2-deoxy-2-[18F]fluoro-D-glucose micro positron emission tomography imaging for efficacy of

new anticancer drugs: a case study with bortezomib in prostate cancer murine model. Mol Imaging Biol 2006;8(5):300–8.

13. Herschman HR. Micro-PET imaging and small animal models of disease. Curr Opin Immunol 2003;15:378–84.

14. Nanni C, Di Leo K, Tonelli R, et al. FDG small animal PET permits early detection of malignant cells in a xenograft murine model. Eur J Nucl Med Mol Imaging 2007;34(5):755–62.

15. Sturm RA. Skin colour and skin cancer: MC1R, the genetic link. Melanoma Res 2002;12:405–16.

16. Siegrist W, Solca F, Stutz S, et al. Characterization of receptors for alphamelanocyte-stimulating hormone on human melanoma cells. Cancer Res 1989;49: 6352–8.

17. Siegrist W, Stutz S, Eberle AN. Homologous and heterologous regulation of alpha-melanocyte-stimulating hormone receptors in human and mouse melanoma cell lines. Cancer Res 1994;54: 2604–10.

18. Vaidyanathan G, Zalutsky MR. Fluorine-18-labeled [Nle4, D-Phe7]-alpha-MSH, an alpha-melanocyte stimulating hormone analogue. Nucl Med Biol 1997;24:171–8.

19. Chen J, Cheng Z, Hoffman TJ, et al. Melanoma-targeting properties of (99m)technetium-labeled cyclic alpha-melanocyte-stimulating hormone peptide analogues. Cancer Res 2000;60:5649–58.

20. Chen J, Giblin MF, Wang N, et al. In vivo evaluation of 99mTc/188Re-labeled linear alpha-melanocyte stimulating hormone analogs for specific melanoma targeting. Nucl Med Biol 1999;26:687–93.

21. Cheng Z, Chen J, Miao Y, et al. Modification of the structure of a metallopeptide: synthesis and biological evaluation of 111In-labeled DOTA-conjugated rhenium-cyclized alpha-MSH analogues. J Med Chem 2002;45:3048–56.

22. Chen J, Cheng Z, Owen NK, et al. Evaluation of an 111In-DOTA-rhenium cyclized alpha-MSH analog: a novel cyclic-peptide analog with improved tumor targeting properties. J Nucl Med 2001;42:1847–55.

23. Froidevaux S, Calame-Christe M, Tanner H, et al. A novel DOTA-alpha-melanocyte-stimulating hormone analog for metastatic melanoma diagnosis. J Nucl Med 2002;43:1699–706.

24. Froidevaux S, Calame-Christe M, Tanner H, et al. Melanoma targeting with DOTA-alpha-melanocyte-stimulating hormone analogs: structural parameters affecting tumor uptake and kidney uptake. J Nucl Med 2005;46:887–95.

25. Bagutti C, Stolz B, Albert R, et al. [111In]-DTPA-labeled analogues of alpha-melanocyte-stimulating hormone for melanoma targeting: receptor binding in vitro and in vivo. Int J Cancer 1994;58:749–55.

26. Bard DR. An improved imaging agent for malignant melanoma, based on [Nle4, D-Phe7]alpha-

melanocyte stimulating hormone. Nucl Med Commun 1995;16:860–6.

27. Cheng Z, Chen J, Quinn TP, et al. Radioiodination of rhenium cyclized alpha-melanocyte-stimulating hormone resulting in enhanced radioactivity localization and retention in melanoma. Cancer Res 2004;64:1411–8.

28. Froidevaux S, Calame-Christe M, Schuhmacher J, et al. A gallium-labeled DOTA-alpha-melanocyte-stimulating hormone analog for PET imaging of melanoma metastases. J Nucl Med 2004;45:116–23.

29. McQuade P, Miao Y, Yoo J, et al. Imaging of melanoma using 64Cu- and 86Y-DOTA-ReCCMSH (Arg11), a cyclized peptide analogue of alpha-MSH. J Med Chem 2005;48:2985–92.

30. Cheng Z, Xiong ZM, Wu Y, et al. MicroPET imaging of melanoma using Cu-64 labeled alpha-melanocyte stimulating hormone peptide analogue. Mol Imaging Biol 2005;7:126.

31. Cheng Z, Xiong ZM, Subbarayan M, et al. 64Cu labeled alphamelanocyte stimulating hormone analog for microPET imaging of melanocortin 1 receptor expression. Bioconjug Chem 2007;18(3): 765–72.

32. Miao Y, Owen NK, Fisher DR, et al. Therapeutic efficacy of a 188Re-labeled alpha-melanocyte-stimulating hormone peptide analog in murine and human melanoma-bearing mouse models. J Nucl Med 2005; 46:121–9.

33. Miao Y, Hylarides M, Fisher DR, et al. Melanoma therapy via peptide-targeted a-radiation. Clin Cancer Res 2005;11:5616–21.

34. Wei L, Zhang X, Gallazzi F, et al. Melanoma imaging using (111)In-, (86)Y- and (68)Ga-labeled CHX-A'-Re(Arg11)CCMSH. Nucl Med Biol 2009; 36(4):345–54.

35. Wei L, Miao Y, Gallazzi F, et al. Gallium-68-labeled DOTA-rhenium-cyclized alpha-melanocyte-stimulating hormone analog for imaging of malignant melanoma. Nucl Med Biol 2007;34(8):945–53.

36. Cheng Z, Zhang L, Graves E, et al. Small-animal PET of melanocortin 1 receptor expression using a 18F-labeled alpha-melanocyte-stimulating hormone analog. J Nucl Med 2007;48(6):987–94.

37. Ren G, Liu Z, Miao Z, et al. PET of malignant melanoma using 18F-labeled metallopeptides. J Nucl Med 2009;50(11):1865–72.

38. Sobal G, Rodrigues M, Sinzinger H. Radioiodinated methylene blue: a promising agent for melanoma scintigraphy–labelling, stability and in vitro uptake by melanoma cells. Anticancer Res 2008; 28:3691–6.

39. Beatovic S, Obradovic V, Latkovic Z, et al. Diagnosis and follow up of primary ocular melanoma by radioimmunoscintigraphy. J BUON 2004;9:299–302.

40. Voss SD, Smith SV, DiBartolo N, et al. Positron emission tomography (PET) imaging of neuroblastoma

and melanoma with 64Cu-SarAr immunoconjugates. Proc Natl Acad Sci U S A 2007;104:17489–93.

41. Kato K, Kubota T, Ikeda M, et al. Low efficacy of 18F-FDG PET for detection of uveal malignant melanoma compared with 123I-IMP SPECT. J Nucl Med 2006; 47:404–9.

42. Guo H, Shenoy N, Gershman BM, et al. Metastatic melanoma imaging with an (111)In-labeled lactam bridge-cyclized alpha-melanocyte-stimulating hormone peptide. Nucl Med Biol 2009;36:267–76.

43. Miao Y, Figueroa SD, Fisher DR, et al. 203Pb-labeled a-melanocyte-stimulating hormone peptide as an imaging probe for melanoma detection. J Nucl Med 2008;49:823–9.

44. Chezal JM, Papon J, Labarre P, et al. Evaluation of radiolabeled (hetero)aromatic analogues of N-(2-diethylaminoethyl)-4-iodobenzamide for imaging and targeted radionuclide therapy of melanoma. J Med Chem 2008;51:3133–44.

45. Pham TQ, Greguric I, Liu X, et al. Synthesis and evaluation of novel radioiodinated benzamides for malignant melanoma. J Med Chem 2007;50:3561–72.

46. Moins N, D'Incan M, Bonafous J, et al. 123I-N-(2-diethylaminoethyl)-2- iodobenzamide: a potential imaging agent for cutaneous melanoma staging. Eur J Nucl Med Mol Imaging 2002;29:1478–84.

47. Sillaire-Houtmann I, Bonafous J, Veyre A, et al. Phase 2 clinical study of 123IN-(2-diethylaminoethyl)-2-iodobenzamide in the diagnostic of primary and metastatic ocular melanoma. J Fr Ophtalmol 2004;27:34–9.

48. Bacin F, Michelot J, Bonafous J, et al. Clinical study of [123I] N-(2-diethylaminoethyl)-4-iodobenzamide in the diagnosis of primary and metastatic ocular melanoma. Acta Ophthalmol Scand 1998;76:56–61.

49. Larisch R, Schulte KW, Vosberg H, et al. Differential accumulation of iodine-123-iodobenzamide in melanotic and amelanotic melanoma metastases in vivo. J Nucl Med 1998;39:996–1001.

50. Greguric I, Taylor SR, Denoyer D, et al. Discovery of [18F]N-(2-(diethylamino) ethyl)-6-fluoronicotinamide: a melanoma positron emission tomography imaging radiotracer with high tumor to body contrast ratio and rapid renal clearance. J Med Chem 2009;52: 5299–302.

51. Denoyer D, Greguric I, Roselt P, et al. High-contrast PET of melanoma using (18)F-MEL050, a selective probe for melanin with predominantly renal clearance. J Nucl Med 2010;51(3):441–7.

52. Ren G, Miao Z, Liu H, et al. Melanin-targeted preclinical PET imaging of melanoma metastasis. J Nucl Med 2009;50(10):1692–9.

53. Boisgard R, Vincent-Naulleau S, Leplat JJ, et al. A new animal model for the imaging of melanoma: correlation of FDG PET with clinical outcome, macroscopic aspect and histological classification in Melanoblastoma-bearing Libechov Minipigs. Eur J Nucl Med Mol Imaging 2003;30(6):826–34.

Ocular Melanoma and Other Unusual Sites

Gaia Grassetto, MD[a],*, David Fuster, MD, PhD[b],
Abass Alavi, MD, PhD(Hon), DSc(Hon)[c],
Domenico Rubello, MD[a]

KEYWORDS

- Noncutaneous melanoma • Ocular melanoma
- Choroid melanoma • Mucous membrane melanoma
- Meningeal melanoma • PET/CT • SPECT
- Nuclear medicine

Melanocytes are melanin-producing dendritic-like cells that derive from the neural crest. Melanocyte precursors migrate especially to the skin (epidermis and dermis) by way of the dorsolateral pathway between the somites and the ectoderm, and in smaller numbers they migrate via the dorso-ventral pathway, between the neural tube and somites, to other sites of the body, including eyes, mucosal sites (respiratory tract, digestive tract, genitourinary tract), and meninges.[1–6]

Malignant transformation of melanocytes generates malignant melanoma, which comprises about 4.3% of all new cancers diagnosed per year in the United States.[7,8] Melanoma can be cutaneous, if it develops from melanocytes of the skin, or noncutaneous, if it develops from nonskin melanocytes. Cutaneous melanoma is the most frequent kind of melanoma, whereas only 4% to 5% of all malignant melanomas arise from an extracutaneous site. Among these, ocular melanoma is the most frequent.[1,6,9]

Although malignant melanoma has currently the fastest increase in incidence among all types of cancer, noncutaneous melanomas remain very rare and it is difficult to determine their real incidence: some investigators report an incidence of about 0.7 new diagnoses per 100,000 per year.[6,9–11] Moreover, noncutaneous melanomas cause considerable diagnostic difficulties, in particular during the preoperative phase, and their histologic separation from other tumor types, especially undifferentiated carcinomas, high-grade sarcomas, and lymphomas, is crucial from both a diagnostic and prognostic point of view.[1] Above all, when the lesions are amelanotic it is often necessary to examine the immunoprofile to establish the malignant nature, assessing the positivity of S-100 protein, HMB45, and vimentin.[1,3,12,13]

Although cutaneous and extracutaneous melanomas arise from the same cell, they differ in some aspects, especially regarding their biologic behavior. Noncutaneous melanomas, especially the ones at mucosal sites, have worse outcome and prognosis than cutaneous melanoma. In fact, generally they are characterized by vascular invasion and tumor necrosis and with early hematogenous dissemination, preferentially to the liver.[1] Nevertheless, it is worth noting that the rarity of these tumors makes their diagnosis more difficult, and it is not uncommon to find metastatic disease at the time of diagnosis. Therefore it is not yet clear whether the poor prognosis is intrinsic to this tumor or whether delay in detection and removal are responsible.[6] Moreover, for staging noncutaneous melanoma it is not possible to use the Clark level and Breslow index, and a standard internationally accepted staging system does not exist.[1,3,7,14–16] The poorer prognosis of noncutaneous melanomas is also caused by the difficulty

[a] Department of Nuclear Medicine, PET/CT Centre, Santa Maria della Misericordia Hospital, Via Tre Martiri 140, 45100 Rovigo, Italy
[b] Nuclear Medicine Department, Hospital Clínic of Barcelona, Villarroel 170, 08036 Barcelona, Spain
[c] Department of Radiology, Hospital of the University of Pennsylvania, 3400 Spruce Street, Philadelphia, PA 19104, USA
* Corresponding author.
E-mail address: gagra57@libero.it

PET Clin 6 (2011) 79–89
doi:10.1016/j.cpet.2011.01.002

in performing extensive resection of the primary lesion, because of its anatomic location, or radical lymphadenectomy.[7] Moreover, the role of adjuvant treatment has not yet been proven.[7]

OCULAR MELANOMA
Epidemiology

Ocular melanoma is the most frequent extracutaneous melanoma, accounting for 80% of these tumors.[1,17,18] Moreover, it is worth noting that ocular melanoma is the most common primary tumor of the eye in the adult (70%) followed by retinoblastoma (13%).[1,19–21] It is more common among white people, with a rate 0 to 10 times higher than in blacks, and is more frequent in men than in women.[1,21–24] In particular, among men 82.7% of noncutaneous melanomas are ocular while among women 65% are ocular.[22]

Ocular melanoma can arise in several parts of the eye where melanocytes are located: the uvea, the vascular middle layer positioned between retina and sclera that can be divided into the front part, which includes the iris and the ciliary body, and the back portion, constituted by the choroid; the stroma layer of the sclera; and the mucosa layer of the conjunctiva.[1,20,25]

The most common site for ocular melanoma is the uvea: 85% of eye melanomas arise from uvea, of which 86.3% occur in the choroid layer.[1,9,19,20,22,23,26,27] Uvea melanoma, which has a reported incidence of 6 in each million people in North America, is rare before the age of 20 years and after age 75, being more frequent between the ages of 55 and 65.[6,19,28–31]

The causes for ocular melanoma are unidentified but some risk factors are known[25]:

Eye color: People with blue eyes show greater probability than people with brown eyes to develop melanoma of the eye.

Genetic disposition: Dysplastic nevus syndrome increases the risk of skin and ocular melanoma. People with oculodermal melanocytosis or nevus of Ota, that is, an abnormal skin pigmentation involving the eyelid and adjacent tissue with increased pigmentation of the uvea, have a higher risk for ocular melanoma. Certain chromosomal abnormalities, such as those on chromosome 3, constitute a risk factor.

Sun exposure: Ultraviolet light causes melanoma of the skin and probably is also associated with ocular melanoma, although this has as yet not been proved.

Older age

White race.

Histology

Macroscopically, ocular melanoma may appear as a mass with variable pigmentation. Microscopically, these tumors are composed of spindle cells and/or epithelioid cells. From a cytologic point of view Callender classification is used, which distinguishes 3 categories of ocular melanoma: spindle cell (A or B type) melanoma, epithelioid cell type melanoma, and mixed forms.[1,19,32] The prognosis is worse for pure epithelioid cell type tumors that show a 5-year survival rate of 25% to 30% versus 90% to 100% for pure spindle A form, 66% to 75% for pure spindle B, and 50% for spindle B/epithelioid.[1,19] Moreover, to differentiate melanoma from other kinds of ocular lesions, as already mentioned it is often necessary to perform immunohistochemistry and demonstrate the melanocytic nature of the cell with positive staining for S-100, HMB45, and vimentin.[1,19] Despite this tool, however, it is not possible to distinguish an ocular metastatic eye lesion from cutaneous melanoma.[19]

Diagnosis

In general, ocular melanoma is asymptomatic, so it can be revealed by routine eye examination.[28] If symptoms appear, they depend on the location of the lesion:

Melanoma of the iris can cause discoloration of the iris itself or a brown spot on the outside of the eye.

Melanomas that develop near the lens can push or tilt the lens itself causing astigmatism with blurring of vision.

Melanoma in the ciliary body generates distortion of the pupil, which can show an irregular shape, and may interfere with accommodation.

Melanoma of the choroid can leak fluid beneath the retina making it detach, causing flashing lights and floating spots. If it originates near the macula it can destroy the fovea, with loss of vision and change in color perception.[1,25,27,28,33]

To diagnose an ocular lesion, usually an ophthalmoscopic examination is necessary. In particular choroidal melanoma, the most frequent malignant lesion of the eye, appears as an irregular, solid, subretinal mass that commonly extends into the retina and vitreous, causing retinal detachment.[1,28] In general, it is pigmented due to the melanin normally produced by melanocytes. However, sometimes the melanocytes lose the ability to make melanin pigment and an amelanotic (nonpigmented) lesion can be found.[28] Another typical diagnostic characteristic is the presence of orange pigment (lipofuscin) on the choroidal melanoma surface, due to cell death on the superficial layer of the lesion.[28]

In more than 96% of cases ocular melanoma can be correctly diagnosed by ophthalmoscopy. Occasionally a biopsy is needed, even if it is preferably avoided because it requires an open procedure, with the risk of letting melanoma cells out, hemorrhage, and infection.[28]

Morphologic Conventional Imaging

After intraocular examination by ophthalmoscopy, eye ultrasonography (US) is mandatory to confirm and characterize the suspected lesion.[19,20,25,27,34] Eye US is useful to differentiate ocular melanoma from other kinds of lesions, that is, metastases or hemangioma, and it is necessary to measure the melanoma size, the most important prognostic factor.[19,33] The most used choroidal melanoma classification, the one proposed by the COMS (Collaborative Ocular Melanoma Study group),[19,35] uses the size of the lesion to separate ocular melanoma into 3 different types with respect to the thickness and the basal diameter of the lesion:

Small-sized choroidal melanoma: 1–2.5 mm thickness; 5 mm basal diameter
Medium-sized choroidal melanoma: 2.5–10 mm thickness; 5–16 mm basal diameter
Large-sized choroidal melanoma: 10 mm thickness; 16 mm basal diameter.

Moreover, other than the tumor shape and dimensions, US can be used to evaluate the internal tumor reflectivity and the association of retina detachment, and it can examine melanoma extension behind the eye into the orbit (extrascleral extension).[28,36–38] Fluorescein angiography and indocyanine green angiography are also useful to confirm the diagnosis and, above all, to differentiate suspected melanoma from other kinds of lesions.[25,34] In particular, angiography offers a unique view of the tumor borders, vascular patterns, and leakage.[36,39]

Using all these procedures and criteria, the accuracy of clinical diagnosis of ocular melanoma is about 99.6%.[36,40,41] In doubtful cases contrast enhancement computed tomography (CT) and magnetic resonance (MR) imaging of the orbit may be helpful in characterizing the nature of the primary lesion and in evaluating the locoregional invasion.[19] Moreover, total-body CT, together with hepatic US, chest radiography, and blood examination, is mandatory in staging the disease and in assessing the presence of metastatic foci.[19] Melanoma of the eye metastasizes preferentially to the liver, but may also spread to the skin, lung, brain, ovary, kidney, and bone.[1,42–49] However, if extraocular tumor extension is present, with invasion of the conjunctival lymphatics, regional lymph node metastasis is also possible.[42,50] In general, lymph node involvement is delayed in advanced stages of disease.[19]

Nuclear Medicine

Functional imaging is not the first choice of examination in ocular melanoma. Nevertheless, it can be helpful in doubtful cases and in staging.

Clinical diagnosis of ocular melanoma is usually done by conventional techniques already described, with an accuracy of greater than 99%. However, if a lesion is not typical the diagnosis becomes more difficult. Above all, lesions accompanied by retinal detachment, cataract, or intravitreous hemorrhage can be misdiagnosed.[21,51]

Furthermore, in some cases, distinguishing a choroidal melanoma in its early stage from a choroidal nevus is not so simple.[21,52] Many radiopharmaceuticals have been evaluated, the most favorable of which for the diagnosis of an ocular melanoma seems to be ^{123}I-IMP (N-isopropyl-p-[^{123}I]iodoamphetamine). This tracer, originally used for cerebral blood flow studies, is accumulated by cells that actively produce melanin and allows single-photon emission CT (SPECT) acquisition.[23,51,53–55] The procedure consists of intravenous injection of 111 to 222 MBq (3–6 mCi) of ^{123}I-IMP and subsequent brain-SPECT acquisition in early and late phases, up until 48 h.[51] Goto[21] has studied 63 patients with untreated ocular lesions with ^{123}I-IMP SPECT, and reported good results: 36 of 63 were negative on ^{123}I-IMP SPECT, and all 36 except for one had histologic confirmation of other ocular lesions different from melanoma (choroidal nevus, hemangioma, metastatic choroidal tumor, and so forth). Twenty-seven of 63 showed high accumulation of the tracer at ocular lesion site, especially in late-phase SPECT. All except 2 patients had uveal melanoma histologically confirmed. Also, Abe and colleagues[51] reported an accuracy of 94.7% for ^{123}I-IMP SPECT and a sensitivity of about 100% on late-phase images (48 hours post infection). Nevertheless, as with any other imaging tool, ^{123}I-IMP SPECT has some drawbacks: amelanotic lesions and ocular melanoma smaller than 4 mm in size can be missed and some nonmelanoma lesions, such as melanin-rich nevus, leiomyoma, metastatic choroidal tumor, uveoscleritis, and adenocarcinoma of the pigment epithelium of ciliary body, can be false-positive.[21,51] Other than ocular melanoma diagnosis, ^{123}I-IMP SPECT seems useful to assess response to treatment after eye-preserving therapy. Sou and colleagues[53] studied 3 patients with choroidal melanoma and followed them for a period of 18 months, from the diagnosis until some months after radiotherapy. These investigators reported that ^{123}I-IMP SPECT gave important information about tumor activity after radiation therapy, and was an alternative tool for assessment of the effect of treatment (usually measured by variation in lesion size with US or MR imaging).

After ocular melanoma diagnosis, the COMS suggests baseline and periodic examinations to look for the presence of metastases: these include physical examination (hepatomegaly, cutaneous and subcutaneous nodularity), liver function tests, and radiographic imaging of the chest. If liver function tests are abnormal, MR imaging or CT of the abdomen followed by biopsy are recommended.[42–44,56,57] Others have recommended a liver screening test with abdominal US.[56,58]

In the last decade, 2-[^{18}F]fluoro-2-deoxy-D-glucose (FDG) PET/CT has become a widely accepted functional imaging modality to diagnose, stage, restage, and evaluate the response to treatment for many types of cancer. This modality is very useful for the detection of primary and metastatic lesions of cutaneous melanoma. However, FDG PET/CT has not been as successful for diagnosing ocular melanoma.[23,41] In fact it is not sensitive enough to detect the primary ocular lesion because of the small tumor size. Moreover, ocular space is characterized by physiologic FDG uptake in normal tissue near the eye, such as ocular muscles and the brain, which can result in suboptimal interpretation of an FDG scan.[23,59] In the study by Reddy and colleagues,[41] only 28% of 50 patients with nontreated choroidal melanoma were FDG-positive and no small-choroidal tumor, as classified by COMS, were detected by FDG PET/CT. Moreover, not all large tumors (medium and large size for COMS classification) were FDG-positive: tumor size is not the only factor governing FDG uptake.[23,36] Therefore, in light of these results, it is not possible to consider FDG PET/CT as a useful tool for differentiating choroidal melanoma from choroidal nevus.[41] Nevertheless, Reddy and colleagues[41] and Finger and colleagues[36] found that with increasing dimension of the lesion, the intensity of uptake (measured by standardized uptake value [SUV]) also increases, and this correlates with the known clinical, pathologic, and ultrasound features linked to metastatic potential of choroidal melanoma. These findings suggest that the higher the SUV, the higher is the probability for choroidal melanoma to metastasize and to have a bad prognosis (**Fig. 1**).

However, FDG PET/CT is an accepted procedure for staging of ocular melanoma, just as for cutaneous melanoma. Correct cancer staging after the diagnosis of eye melanoma is crucial because it guides the treatment plan and determines the patient's prognosis. FDG PET/CT is a technique that can assess the entire body from vertex to the bottom of the feet for staging

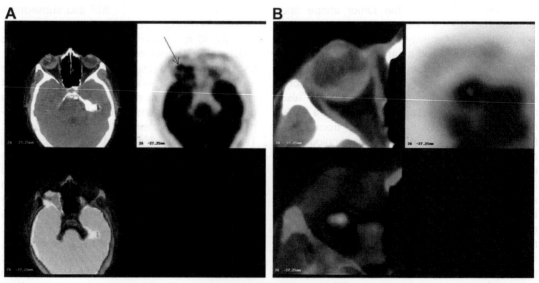

Fig. 1. (A) Right eye choroidal melanoma detected at FDG PET/CT; SUV$_{max}$ = 5.4. Upper left: transaxial CT view. Upper right: transaxial PET view (*arrow* indicates the melanoma). Lower left: transaxial PET/CT fusion view. (B) Detailed imaging of FDG PET/CT of a right eye choroidal melanoma.

purposes. Moreover, coregistration of CT images allows one to fuse PET images on anatomic scans to better localize FDG-positive findings and to increase the specificity of the procedure.

Some investigators, such as the COMS group, reported that despite the high specificity of liver US, liver function tests, and chest radiography, they have low sensitivity in the diagnosis of metastatic uveal melanoma.[56,57,60] It is not uncommon to find liver metastases despite normal liver function tests.[42,56] Using FDG PET/CT as an important examination permits an evaluation of the entire body with a single procedure, and thereafter one could use regional assessments (ie, liver MR imaging) to confirm PET findings. Finger colleagues[56] and Kurli and colleagues[42] studied respectively 52 and 20 patients with untreated choroidal melanoma, using FDG PET/CT.[42,56] Both studies confirmed the important role of FDG PET/CT in ocular melanoma for staging purposes, particularly in patients with large choroidal melanoma without pain, in whom enucleation of the eye can be avoided if widespread disease is discovered. Moreover, the finding of extrahepatic disease may obviate the need for surgical resection and chemotherapy perfusion of the liver. In fact, it is worth noting that up to 75% of patients with metastatic eye melanoma have multiple sites of involvement, mostly in the liver and on bone.[30,57,61] Therefore the treatment plan may be altered and shifted from local treatment to systemic palliative therapy.[30] FDG PET/CT may thus be a cost-effective procedure because it eliminates unnecessary treatment if the disease is widespread.[56]

Using FDG PET/CT to stage melanoma of the eye, is not uncommon to find a second primary cancer. In fact, it is known that cancer patients have twice the risk of developing another cancer than cancer-free patients. Chin and colleagues[30] investigated 139 patients with uveal melanoma: 93 were scanned by FDG PET/CT before treatment and 46 during follow-up. Of all 139 patients 4.3%, in the absence of any symptoms, had second primary, 50% synchronous and 50% metachronous. The investigators showed that FDG PET/CT is more effective in finding second primary cancer than conventional imaging examinations.[30] The same results were also reported for different types of cancer by Choi and colleagues[62]: 4.8% of 547 cancer patients had synchronous primary diagnosed only by FDG PET scan.

Therapy

The choice of treatment depends on the overall stage of the disease.

In particular, if the melanoma is confined to the uvea, the therapy is contingent on the size of the lesion according to COMS classification.[19] For small-sized choroidal melanoma it is possible to choose a "wait and see" approach by US follow-up every 3 months; but when a growth is documented, local treatment is necessary. Nowadays there is a trend toward early treatment of small lesions, and transpupillary thermotherapy seems useful. In particular, some investigators reported complete tumor control without recurrence in 91% of cases after a mean of 3 treatment sessions.[6,63]

For medium-sized melanoma, ^{125}I brachytherapy administered via episcleral plaques is the mainstay of primary therapy, and is preferred to surgical treatment (enucleation). In fact, COMS randomized study results suggest that plaque radiation therapy and enucleation are equally effective for the prevention of metastatic choroidal melanoma. In particular, 5-year survival rate (about 80%) and percentage of subjects who developed metastatic disease (about 10%) are similar for both therapies.[6,19,28,64] Instead of enucleation, radiation therapy allows preservation of the eye and maintenance of good visual acuity in 50% of cases.[19,65,66] Also, radiation therapy with charged particles (helium ion or proton beam) is well supported by long-term follow-up studies[6,67,68] and seems to give the same results as brachytherapy: complete local control in 90% to 95% of cases.[19,69,70]

Large-sized ocular melanomas generally are treated with enucleation. The use of neoadjuvant radiotherapy before surgery was not supported by the results of a COMS study on more than 1000 patients.[6,71] Radiosurgery with the Gamma Knife seems to have a potential role, but other studies are necessary.[6,72]

In cases of metastatic disease the prognosis is very poor, similar to that for advanced cutaneous melanoma; the only treatment with palliative intent is chemotherapeutic drugs and interferon-α.[19]

Prognosis and Outcome

The most important prognostic factors for ocular melanoma are the size of primary lesion and its histologic type: the prognosis is better for small-sized ocular melanoma (COMS classification) and for pure spindle A cells (Callender classification). Patients with small tumors have a low death risk with a 5-year mortality rate of 6%.[6,35] By contrast, the 5-year survival rate of patients with large choroidal melanoma is about 60% with median survival of 7.4 years.[6,71,73]

The mortality rate of ocular melanoma depends on overall stage and the presence of metastases.[19,74] The mortality peak is after 2 to 3 years from ocular enucleation (surgical removal of the eye). Survival rate after 5, 10, and 15 years after enucleation is 65%, 52%, and 46%, respectively.[19,75]

UNUSUAL SITE MELANOMA
Mucosal Melanoma

Other than the ocular site, noncutaneous melanoma can occur in many different mucous membranes. In fact it is common to find melanocytes as normal residents in the mucous membranes of the upper aerodigestive tract (head and neck district), and the gastrointestinal and urogenital tracts.[1] As already mentioned, malignant mucosal melanomas are very rare tumors, comprising about 1% of all malignant melanomas.[76] The first to describe a mucosal melanoma was Weber, in Germany in 1856, and the first to recognize this tumor as a distinct clinical entity was Lucke in 1869.[1,76] Compared with ocular melanomas, the mucosal ones are more frequent in populations where incidence of skin melanoma is low (non-Caucasians). Moreover, because of their rarity and their poorly visible location, their diagnosis is generally delayed until the advanced stages of disease. Therefore, mucosal melanomas have generally a worse prognosis then cutaneous melanoma: the 5-year survival rates are lower than 50%.[1,6,76,77] The worse prognosis is caused by the frequent microscopic blood vessel and lymphatic invasion, which contributes to their aggressive behavior.[6,78]

It is worth noting that a primary mucosal melanoma is indistinguishable from mucous membrane metastasis of cutaneous melanoma, so the diagnosis of extracutaneous malignant melanoma can be made only by detecting both typical and atypical melanocytes on the edges of the lesions.[6]

A uniform international classification system does not exist. Nevertheless, the United States National Institutes of Health has proposed a classification system according to clinical stage[6,79]:

Stage 1: Localized primary malignant melanoma
Stage 2: Local recurrence
Stage 3: Regional lymph node metastases
Stage 4: Distant metastases.

As already mentioned, it is not possible to use Clark level and Breslow index for a prognostic evaluation of mucosal melanoma; however, there seems to be a correlation between the depth of lesion and its outcome.[6]

Head and Neck Mucosal Melanoma

Half of malignant mucosal melanomas arise from the head and neck region, especially in nasal and paranasal sinuses (56% of head and neck mucosal melanomas) and oral cavity (44% of head and neck mucosal melanomas).[6,76,80,81] The third most frequent location is a pharyngolaryngeal site.[6] These melanomas usually occur in older patients, between their sixth and eighth decades of life, without sex predilection.[1]

About 50% of head and neck mucosal melanomas show metastatic disease at presentation, especially the ones originating in the oral cavity that disseminate early to regional lymph nodes.[6,81] These tumors therefore usually have a bad prognosis, with a 5-year survival rate of between 20% and 45%.[6,81,82]

The symptoms of head and neck mucosal melanoma depend on lesion location. Melanomas of nasal cavity, paranasal sinus, and nasopharynx manifest themselves very late with few symptoms such as epistaxis, mass, nasal obstruction and, less often, minimal pain.[6] Melanomas of the oral cavity generally develop from the keratinized mucosa overlying the maxilla: 50% from hard palate, 26% from alveolar ridge, and 8% from soft palate.[83] Less frequently they can arise from the lips, the buccal mucous membrane, the floor of the mouth, and the tongue.[6] The tumors are usually asymptomatic, with only a pigmented lesion that sometimes can cause dental and chewing difficulties.[6] Nevertheless, 33% of head and neck mucosal melanomas have an amelanotic appearance that results in delayed diagnosis.[76] Because of their delayed discovery, nearly 50% of mucosal head and neck melanomas, especially the oral ones, have lymph node metastasis at diagnosis, and 20% have widespread disease.[83] Among mucosal melanomas those of the oral cavity appear to have the worst prognosis, with a 5-year survival rate of 5%.[83] Some benign lesions that simulate oral mucosal melanoma include mucosal melanotic macule and labial melanotic macule.[83] Thus, in light of the bad prognosis of mucosal melanoma it is advisable to excise all pigmented oral mucosal lesions, even those with benign appearance.[83]

The treatment of choice is surgery because it is the only potentially curative treatment.[6] Prophylactic neck node dissection is not recommended, because head and neck tumors metastasize to regional lymph nodes less frequently than squamous carcinomas in the same region.[76] However, in some cases neck node dissection may prolong the survival period, but some investigators consider it sufficient to extirpate only the clinically positive lymph nodes.[6] The value of elective neck dissection remains doubtful, as is the role of sentinel lymph node biopsy.[6] The role of radiation and chemo-/immunotherapy is not clear. Radiation is recommended as a palliative measure for recurrence, but its value as adjuvant treatment after surgery is unproven.[6,76] Chemo-/immunotherapy is generally used with adjuvant or palliative intention.[76,82]

Urogenital Tract Mucosal Melanoma

This kind of melanoma is prevalent in women, in whom the most frequent location is the vulva, especially labia majora, followed by vagina and, very rarely, cervix, ovaries, and uterus.[6,83] These tumors are highly aggressive and they are often confused with poorly differentiated carcinomas.[1] At diagnosis most of these tumors are more than 2 mm thick. The reported survival rate for vulvar primary varies from 27% to 59%, and that for vagina primary is 13% to 33%.[6] Symptoms are often bleeding, discharge, itching, feeling of mass, urinary disturbance, inguinal swelling, and pain.[1,6] Surgical excision is the mainstay of therapy and when the primary melanoma spreads to the urethra or rectum, an anterior or posterior exenteration is needed.[6] Prophylactic node dissection is also under debate: some investigators suggest the inguinofemoral lymphadenectomy at the time of primary surgery only in cases of clinically positive lymph nodes.[6] Sentinel lymph node biopsy seems feasible in vulvar and vaginal melanomas, and some investigators suggest avoiding inguinofemoral lymphadenectomy if sentinel node biopsy is negative.[6]

The most common location in the urinary tract is the distal urethra including the fossa navicularis and urethral meatus.[6] Associated symptoms are usually mass, hematuria, dysuria, decreased urinary flow, and bleeding.[6] These tumors are very rare but very malignant, with a poor prognosis due to their tendency to locally invade the corpus cavernosus in men and the vulva and vagina in women.[1] Surgery is the mainstay of therapy, and includes local excision for confined lesions and extensive urethrectomy (two-thirds of the urethra in women and amputation of the penis in men with perineal urethrostomy) for locally advanced tumors, together with inguinal lymphadenectomy and radiotherapy.[1]

Gastrointestinal Tract Mucosal Melanoma

These tumors represent about 1.5% to 2% of all melanomas. Their most frequent locations are anorectum, esophagus, and gallbladder.[1]

The anorectal presentation is the third most frequent form of malignant melanoma after skin and ocular, and comprises 0.25% to 1.25% of malignancies originating in the anorectal region.[1,6] The majority develop from melanocytes of the anal squamous zone distal to the dentate line.[1] Anorectal melanomas do not have sex predilection and have no correlation with sun exposure; they are more frequent in the sixth and seventh decades of life and in AIDS patients.[1] Anorectal melanomas manifest themselves by anal bleeding, painful defecation, and a pigmented or nonpigmented polypoid mass prolapsing through the anus like hemorrhoids.[1] An example of rectal melanoma well depicted at FDG PET/CT is shown in **Fig. 2**. More than half of these patients have widespread disease at diagnosis, at both inguinal and iliac lymph nodes, due to rich lymphatics of the anal zone and at liver, lung, bone, and other organs by hematogenous dissemination.[1,83] The prognosis is generally very poor (5-year survival rate of 10%) and correlates with the thickness of the lesion: tumors with thickness less than 2 mm have a better prognosis (15% vs 10% survival rate).[1,83] There is no agreement about the treatment of these mucosal melanomas It is worth noting that about 90% of patients die regardless of surgical approach or adjuvant therapy.[1]

Melanoma can also arise from esophagus mucosa where melanocytes are normally present. It is a very rare tumor comprising 0.1% to 0.2% of all esophagus malignancies.[1] This melanoma is more common in men and occurs after the sixth decade of life. Usually it presents with dysphagia, weight loss, pain, and melena.[1] Nearly 50% of patients have metastases at diagnosis, especially in regional lymph nodes, lung, pleura, and liver.[1] The prognosis is poor and the reported 5-year survival rate ranges from 4.2% to 37%.[6] Surgical resection en bloc with lymph node dissection is the treatment of choice.[1] Radiotherapy and chemotherapy usually have palliative intent.[6]

Primary melanoma of the gallbladder is very rare (30 cases are reported in the literature).[1] Because 50% of all metastatic tumors affecting the gallbladder are melanoma, it can be difficult to differentiate primary melanoma from metastasis. For this reason, it is important to indentify typical and atypical melanocytes at the edge of the lesion and assess the presence of junctional component with clusters of melanocytes at the mucosal/submucosal junction adjacent to the area of tumor mass.[6] The principal symptoms are acute cholecystitis, obstructive jaundice, pain, and melena.[6] Surgery is also the mainstay of therapy for this kind of melanoma.

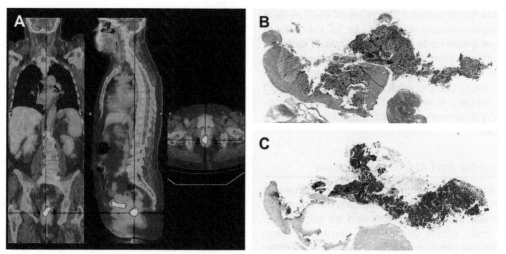

Fig. 2. (*A*) Large rectum melanoma shown on FDG PET/CT; SUV$_{max}$ = 10.3. Left: fusion PET/CT coronal view. Middle: fusion PET/CT sagittal view. Right: fusion PET/CT transaxial view. (*B*) Immunohistochemical analysis of the rectal lesion by hematoxylin and eosin staining (original magnification factor 1:100). (*C*) Immunohistochemical analysis of the rectal lesion by Melan A (MART-1), a specific marker of melanocytes (original magnification factor 1:100).

Meningeal Melanoma

Other than mucous membrane, another unusual site of melanoma is the meninges.[6] Whereas brain metastases from skin melanoma are very frequent, primary intracranial melanoma account for only 1% of all melanoma. More often they arise from leptomeninges (arachnoidea mater and pia mater) and rarely from dura mater.[6] The symptoms depend on the location and include aphasia, dysarthria, hemiparesis, declining cognitive functions, diplopia, ataxia, facial paresis, and so forth. Moreover, more general symptoms such as headache may be present.[6] Meningeal melanoma rarely metastasizes outside the brain, but usually recurs locally and may spread along the meninges.[6] Meningeal melanoma must be differentiated from meningeal melanocytoma, which is a benign lesion that develops from melanocytes of the leptomeninges in the posterior fossa or in the upper spinal cord in adults.[6] Of course, preoperative discrimination is impossible but total resection is the therapy for both types of lesions.[6] Solitary meningeal melanoma is more frequent in adults and has a slightly better prognosis than diffuse meningeal melanoma. This condition preferentially afflicts children with a mean age of 5 years and is associated with a rare phakomatosis or neurocutaneous melanosis. Its prognosis is very poor, with a mean survival of 6.7 months versus 20.7 months for solitary meningeal melanoma.[6] Diffuse meningeal melanoma appears with increasing intracranial pressure secondary to tumoral obliteration of the basal cisterns. Surgical insertion of shunt reduces intracranial pressure, with only palliative intent.[6]

The authors have not found any studies that evaluate the usefulness of nuclear medicine techniques in mucous membrane and meningeal melanoma. FDG PET/CT may have a potential role in the staging of mucous membrane melanoma. FDG PET/CT would be very helpful to determine the stage of disease so as to avoid unnecessary surgery. However, for meningeal melanoma one cannot predict the efficacy of FDG PET/CT because of the physiologically high uptake of this agent in brain structures.

Nevertheless, to evaluate the future role of functional imaging, especially that of FDG PET/CT imaging, in noncutaneous melanoma, further investigation is needed.

REFERENCES

1. Hussein MR. Extracutaneous malignant melanomas. Cancer Invest 2008;26(5):516–34.
2. Hussein MR. Genetic pathways to melanoma tumorigenesis. J Clin Pathol 2004;57(8):797–801.
3. Hussein MR, Haemel AK, Albert DM, et al. Microsatellite instability and alterations of mismatch repair protein expression in choroidal melanomas. Arch Ophthalmol 2005;123(12):1705–11.
4. Cheung M, Briscoe J. Neural crest development is regulated by the transcription factor Sox9. Development 2003;130(23):5681–93.
5. Faas L, Rovasio RA. Distribution patterns of neural-crest-derived melanocyte precursor cells in the quail embryo. Anat Rec 1998;251(2):200–6.
6. Thoelke A, Willrodt S, Hauschild A, et al. Primary extracutaneous malignant melanoma: a comprehensive

review with emphasis on treatment. Onkologie 2004; 27(5):492–9.

7. Kim HS, Kim EK, Jun HJ, et al. Noncutaneous malignant melanoma: a prognostic model from a retrospective multicenter study. BMC Cancer 2010;10:167.

8. Jemal A, Siegel R, Ward E, et al. Cancer statistics, 2008. CA Cancer J Clin 2008;58(2):71–96.

9. Chang AE, Karnell LH, Menck HR. The National Cancer Data Base report on cutaneous and noncutaneous melanoma: a summary of 84,836 cases from the past decade. The American College of Surgeons Commission on Cancer and the American Cancer Society. Cancer 1998;83(8):1664–78.

10. Peter RU, Landthaler M, Braun-Falco O. Extracutaneous malignant melanomas: clinical aspects and biology. Hautarzt 1992;43(9):535–41.

11. Krasnow AZ, Elgazzar A. Lymphoscintigraphy. In: Elgazzar A, editor. The pathophysiologic basis of nuclear medicine. Heidelberg (Germany): Springer; 2001. p. 330–7.

12. Hussein MR, Al-Sabae TM, Georgis MN. Analysis of Bcl-2 and p53 protein expression in non-Hodgkin's lymphoma. Ann Oncol 2004;15(12):1849–50.

13. Hussein MR, Al-Sabae TM, Georgis MN. Analysis of the Bcl-2 and p53 protein expression in the lymphoproliferative lesions in the upper Egypt. Cancer Biol Ther 2005;4(3):324–8.

14. Hussein MR, Sun M, Tuthill RJ, et al. Comprehensive analysis of 112 melanocytic skin lesions demonstrates microsatellite instability in melanomas and dysplastic nevi, but not in benign nevi. J Cutan Pathol 2001;28(7):343–50.

15. Hussein MR. The relationships between p53 protein expression and the clinicopathological features in the uveal melanomas. Cancer Biol Ther 2005;4(1): 57–9.

16. Hussein MR, Elsers DA, Fadel SA, et al. Clinicopathological features of melanocytic skin lesions in Egypt. Eur J Cancer Prev 2006;15(1):64–8.

17. Reader S, Grigg J, Billson FA. Choroidal melanoma: a review of the experience of the Sydney eye hospital professorial unit 1979–1995. Aust N Z J Ophthalmol 1997;25(1):15–24.

18. Everaert H, Bossuyt A, Flamen P, et al. Visualizing ocular melanoma using iodine-123-N-(2-diethylaminoethyl)4-iodobenzamide SPECT. J Nucl Med 1997;38(6):870–3.

19. Bajetta E. Melanoma. Guidelines 2009. AIOM (Italian association of medical oncology).

20. MedlinePlus. Melanoma of the eye. 2009. Available at: http://www.nlm.nih.gov/medlineplus/ency/article/001022.htm. Accessed November 14, 2010.

21. Goto H. Clinical efficacy of ^{123}I-IMP SPECT for the diagnosis of malignant uveal melanoma. Int J Clin Oncol 2004;9(2):74–8.

22. McLaughlin CC, Wu XC, Jemal A, et al. Incidence of noncutaneous melanomas in the U.S. Cancer 2005; 103(5):1000–7.

23. Kato K, Kubota T, Ikeda M, et al. Low efficacy of ^{18}F-FDG PET for detection of uveal malignant melanoma compared with ^{123}I-IMP SPECT. J Nucl Med 2006; 47(3):404–9.

24. Singh AD, Topham A. Incidence of uveal melanoma in the United States: 1973–1997. Ophthalmology 2003;110(5):956–61.

25. Mayo Clinic Staff. Eye melanoma. 2008. Available at: http://www.nlm.nih.gov/medlineplus/melanoma.html. Accessed November 14, 2010.

26. Marucci L, Ancukiewicz M, Lane AM, et al. Uveal melanoma recurrence after fractionated proton beam therapy: comparison of survival in patients treated with reirradiation or with enucleation. Int J Radiat Oncol Biol Phys 2011;79(3):842–6.

27. National Cancer Institute. Intraocular (Eye) melanoma treatment. 2008. Available at: http://www.cancer.gov. Accessed November 14, 2010.

28. Eyecancernetwork. Choroidal melanoma. 2010. Available at: http://www.eyecancer.com. Accessed November 14, 2010.

29. Anastassiou G, Tschentscher F, Zeschnigk M. Prognostically relevant markers of malignant melanoma of the uvea. Ophthalmologe 2002;99(5):327–32.

30. Chin K, Finger PT, Kurli M, et al. Second cancers discovered by (18)FDG PET/CT imaging for choroidal melanoma. Optometry 2007;78(8):396–401.

31. Egan KM, Seddon JM, Glynn RJ, et al. Epidemiologic aspects of uveal melanoma. Surv Ophthalmol 1988;32(4):239–51.

32. McLean IW, Foster WD, Zimmerman LE, et al. Modifications of Callender's classification of uveal melanoma at the Armed Forces Institute of Pathology. Am J Ophthalmol 1983;96(4):502–9.

33. Van Gool CA, Thijssen JM, Verbeek AM. B-mode echography of choroidal melanoma; echographic and histological aspects of choroidal excavation. Int Ophthalmol 1991;15(5):327–34.

34. American Cancer Society. Diagnosing melanoma of the eye. 2009. Available at: http://www.cancer.org. Accessed November 14, 2010.

35. Collaborative Ocular Melanoma Study Group. Mortality in patients with small choroidal melanoma. COMS report no. 4. The Collaborative Ocular Melanoma Study Group. Arch Ophthalmol 1997;115(7):886–93.

36. Finger PT, Chin K, Iacob CE. 18-Fluorine-labelled 2-deoxy-2-fluoro-D-glucose positron emission tomography/computed tomography standardised uptake values: a non-invasive biomarker for the risk of metastasis from choroidal melanoma. Br J Ophthalmol 2006;90(10):1263–6.

37. Collaborative Ocular Melanoma Study Group. Echography (Ultrasound) Procedures for the Collaborative Ocular Melanoma Study (COMS), Report no. 12, Part II. J Ophthalmic Nurs Technol 1999;18(5):219–32.

38. Romero JM, Finger PT, Iezzi R, et al. Three-dimensional ultrasonography of choroidal melanoma:

extrascleral extension. Am J Ophthalmol 1998; 126(6):842–4.

39. Oosterhuis JA, van Waveren CW. Fluorescein photography in malignant melanoma. Ophthalmologica 1968;156:101–16.

40. Collaborative Ocular Melanoma Study Group. Accuracy of diagnosis of choroidal melanomas in the Collaborative Ocular Melanoma Study. COMS report no. 1. Arch Ophthalmol 1990;108(9):1268–73.

41. Reddy S, Kurli M, Tena LB, et al. PET/CT imaging: detection of choroidal melanoma. Br J Ophthalmol 2005;89(10):1265–9.

42. Kurli M, Reddy S, Tena LB, et al. Whole body positron emission tomography/computed tomography staging of metastatic choroidal melanoma. Am J Ophthalmol 2005;140(2):193–9.

43. Folberg R. Tumor progression in ocular melanomas. J Invest Dermatol 1993;100(3):326S–31S.

44. Einhorn LH, Burgess MA, Gottlieb JA. Metastatic patterns of choroidal melanoma. Cancer 1974; 34(4):1001–4.

45. Albert DM, Ryan LM, Borden EC. Metastatic ocular and cutaneous melanoma: a comparison of patient characteristics and prognosis. Arch Ophthalmol 1996;114(1):107–8.

46. Gragoudas ES, Egan KM, Seddon JM, et al. Survival of patients with metastases from uveal melanoma. Ophthalmology 1991;98(3):383–9 [discussion: 390].

47. Kath R, Hayungs J, Bornfeld N, et al. Prognosis and treatment of disseminated uveal melanoma. Cancer 1993;72(7):2219–23.

48. Char DH. Metastatic choroidal melanoma. Am J Ophthalmol 1978;86(1):76–80.

49. Flaherty LE, Unger JM, Liu PY, et al. Metastatic melanoma from intraocular primary tumors: the Southwest Oncology Group experience in phase II advanced melanoma clinical trials. Am J Clin Oncol 1998;21(6):568–72.

50. Dithmar S, Diaz CE, Grossniklaus HE. Intraocular melanoma spread to regional lymph nodes: report of two cases. Retina 2000;20(1):76–9.

51. Abe K, Sasaki M, Koga H, et al. Clinical role of ^{123}I-IMP SPECT for the differential diagnosis of ocular malignant melanoma: a time-course analysis. Nucl Med Commun 2007;28(7):567–73.

52. Shields CL, Shields JA. Clinical features of small choroidal melanoma. Curr Opin Ophthalmol 2002; 13(3):135–41.

53. Sou R, Oku N, Ohguro N, et al. The clinical role of N-isopropyl-p-[123I]-iodoamphetamine single photon emission computed tomography in the follow-up of choroidal melanoma after radiotherapy. Jpn J Ophthalmol 2004;48(1):54–8.

54. Holman BL, Wick MM, Kaplan ML, et al. The relationship of the eye uptake of N-isopropyl-p-[123I] iodoamphetamine to melanin production. J Nucl Med 1984;25(3):315–9.

55. Winchell HS, Baldwin RM, Lin TH. Development of I-123-labeled amines for brain studies: localization of I-123 iodophenylalkyl amines in rat brain. J Nucl Med 1980;21(10):940–6.

56. Finger PT, Kurli M, Reddy S, et al. Whole body PET/CT for initial staging of choroidal melanoma. Br J Ophthalmol 2005;89(10):1270–4.

57. Diener-West M, Reynolds SM, Agugliaro DJ, et al. Screening for metastasis from choroidal melanoma: the Collaborative Ocular Melanoma Study Group Report 23. J Clin Oncol 2004;22(12):2438–44.

58. Eskelin S, Pyrhönen S, Summanen P, et al. Screening for metastatic malignant melanoma of the uvea revisited. Cancer 1999;85(5):1151–9.

59. Uren RF, Howman-Giles RB, Thompson JF. Melanoma. In: Aktolun C, Tauxe WN, editors. Nuclear oncology. Heidelberg (Germany): Springer; 1999. p. 59–74.

60. Hicks C, Foss AJ, Hungerford JL. Predictive power of screening tests for metastasis in uveal melanoma. Eye (Lond) 1998;12(Pt 6):945–8.

61. Finger PT, Kurli M, Wesley P, et al. Whole body PET/CT imaging for detection of metastatic choroidal melanoma. Br J Ophthalmol 2004;88(8):1095–7.

62. Choi JY, Lee KS, Kwon OJ, et al. Improved detection of second primary cancer using integrated [^{18}F] fluorodeoxyglucose positron emission tomography and computed tomography for initial tumor staging. J Clin Oncol 2005;23(30):7654–9.

63. Shields CL, Shields JA, Perez N, et al. Primary transpupillary thermotherapy for small choroidal melanoma in 256 consecutive cases: outcomes and limitations. Ophthalmology 2002;109(2):225–34.

64. Diener-West M, Earle JD, Fine SL, et al. The COMS randomized trial of iodine 125 brachytherapy for choroidal melanoma, III: initial mortality findings. COMS Report No. 18. Arch Ophthalmol 2001; 119(7):969–82.

65. Melia BM, Abramson DH, Albert DM, et al. Collaborative ocular melanoma study (COMS) randomized trial of I-125 brachytherapy for medium choroidal melanoma. I. Visual acuity after 3 years COMS report no. 16. Ophthalmology 2001;108(2):348–66.

66. Jampol LM, Moy CS, Murray TG, et al. The COMS randomized trial of iodine 125 brachytherapy for choroidal melanoma: IV. Local treatment failure and enucleation in the first 5 years after brachytherapy. COMS report no. 19. Ophthalmology 2002;109(12):2197–206.

67. Egger E, Zografos L, Schalenbourg A, et al. Eye retention after proton beam radiotherapy for uveal melanoma. Int J Radiat Oncol Biol Phys 2003; 55(4):867–80.

68. Robertson DM. Changing concepts in the management of choroidal melanoma. Am J Ophthalmol 2003;136(1):161–70.

69. Char DH, Kroll SM, Castro J. Ten-year follow-up of helium ion therapy for uveal melanoma. Am J Ophthalmol 1998;125(1):81–9.

70. Gragoudas ES, Lane AM, Munzenrider J, et al. Long-term risk of local failure after proton therapy for choroidal/ciliary body melanoma. Trans Am Ophthalmol Soc 2002;100:43–8 [discussion: 48–9].

71. Collaborative Ocular Melanoma Study Group. The Collaborative Ocular Melanoma Study (COMS) randomized trial of pre-enucleation radiation of large choroidal melanoma II: initial mortality findings. COMS report no. 10. Am J Ophthalmol 1998; 125(6):779–96.

72. Mueller AJ, Schaller U, Talies S, et al. Stereotactic radiosurgery using the Gamma Knife for large uveal melanomas. Ophthalmologe 2003;100(2):122–8.

73. Collaborative Ocular Melanoma Study Group. Assessment of metastatic disease status at death in 435 patients with large choroidal melanoma in the Collaborative Ocular Melanoma Study (COMS): COMS report no. 15. Arch Ophthalmol 2001; 119(5):670–6.

74. Diener-West M, Hawkins BS, Markowitz JA, et al. A review of mortality from choroidal melanoma. II. A meta-analysis of 5-year mortality rates following enucleation, 1966 through 1988. Arch Ophthalmol 1992;110(2):245–50.

75. McCurdy J, Gamel J, McLean I. A simple, efficient, and reproducible method for estimating the malignant potential of uveal melanoma from routine H & E slides. Pathol Res Pract 1991; 187(8):1025–7.

76. Lengyel E, Gilde K, Remenár E, et al. Malignant mucosal melanoma of the head and neck. Pathol Oncol Res 2003;9(1):7–12.

77. Wu E, Golitz LE. Primary noncutaneous melanoma. Clin Lab Med 2000;20:731–4.

78. Tomicic J, Wanebo J II. Mucosal melanomas. Surg Clin North Am 2003;83:237–52.

79. Iversen K, Robins RE. Mucosal malignant melanomas. Am J Surg 1980;139:660–4.

80. Batsakis JD, Regezi JA, Solomon AR, et al. The pathology of head and neck tumors—part 13: mucosal melanoma. Head Neck Surg 1982;4: 404–12.

81. Patel SG, Prasad ML, Escrig M, et al. Primary mucosal malignant melanoma of the head and neck. Head Neck 2002;24:247–57.

82. Guzzo M, Grandi C, Licitra L, et al. Mucosal malignant melanoma of head and neck: forty-eight cases treated at Istituto Nazionale Tumori of Milan. Eur J Surg Oncol 1993;19:316–9.

83. Rogers RS, Gibson LE. Mucosal, Genital, and unusual clinical variants of melanoma. Mayo Clin Proc 1997;72:362–6.

Other PET Tracers and Prospects for the Future

David Fuster, MD, PhD[a],*, Francesca Pons, MD, PhD[a],
Domenico Rubello, MD[b], Abass Alavi, MD, PhD(Hon), DSc(Hon)[c]

KEYWORDS

- PET • Melanoma • α-Melanocyte-stimulating hormone
- Melanin • Nicotinamide • Neoangiogenesis
- Hypoxia tracers

The preliminary diagnosis of malignant melanoma is usually made by visual analysis of a skin lesion, and if this diagnosis is confirmed histologically, complete surgical removal of the lesion, with wide margins, is mandatory. Currently, fludeoxyglucose F 18 (^{18}F FDG) PET, preferably combined with computed tomography, is particularly useful in the diagnosis of advanced disease, notably for its ability to detect visceral, deep soft tissue, and lymph node metastases. However, for the initial assessment of early-stage malignant melanoma, ^{18}F FDG-PET has only a low sensitivity, and in the presence of inflammatory conditions, this tracer also lacks specificity. ^{18}F FDG-PET has proved useful as an independent predictor of chemotherapy response in the management of a variety of malignant tumors.[1] The response rate in most cases of disseminated melanoma is poor, and treatment increasingly needs to be individualized to optimize results. Eisenhauer and colleagues[2] from the Response Evaluation Criteria in Solid Tumors (RECIST) Working Group, when developing RECIST 1.1, considered that there is still not sufficient evidence or standardization to abandon anatomic assessment of tumor burden. However, they consider ^{18}F FDG-PET imaging as a promising adjunct to determine progression of the disease.[2]

There is an urgent need for more-specific tracers to increase the effectiveness of PET for the early detection of melanoma and in the assessment of treatment response. To date, no compounds other than FDG have been approved for use in clinical practice for detection of melanomas, but published studies using other tracers have tried, mainly with murine models as part of research projects, to improve the results of PET in such patients. Most of these studies investigate the potential role of other radiotracers by analyzing the receptor status, hypoxia, and neoangiogenesis phenomenon in the diagnosis, characterization, staging, and treatment protocols of melanoma. In the not-too-distant future, it is hoped that developments and experience with these new agents will provide us with greater certainty in the management of this unpredictable and lethal type of skin cancer. Several PET radiotracers other than FDG are being evaluated for use in melanoma imaging (**Table 1**).

MONOCLONAL ANTIBODIES AGAINST MELANOMA-ASSOCIATED ANTIGENS

Radiolabeled monoclonal antibodies are widely used in nuclear medicine oncology, and interest in this field has increased because of recent

[a] Nuclear Medicine Department, Hospital Clínic of Barcelona, Villarroel 170, 08036 Barcelona, Spain
[b] Department of Nuclear Medicine, PET/CT Center, Santa Maria della Misericordia Hospital, Via Tre Martiri 140, 45100, Rovigo, Italy
[c] Department of Radiology, Hospital of the University of Pennsylvania, 3400 Spruce Street, Philadelphia, PA 19104, USA
* Corresponding author.
E-mail address: dfuster@clinic.ub.es

PET Clin 6 (2011) 91–97
doi:10.1016/j.cpet.2010.12.001
1556-8598/11/$ – see front matter © 2011 Elsevier Inc. All rights reserved.

Table 1
Main developing fields in melanoma using PET tracers other than FDG

Field	References	Radiotracer	Indication
Monoclonal Antibodies	Voss et al[4]	^{64}Cu-SarAr	Anti-GD2 expression
α-MSH	Froidevaux et al[5]	^{68}Ga-DOTA	Tumor retention
	Cheng et al[6]	^{64}Cu-DOTA-NAPamide	Therapy
	McQuade et al[7]	(^{86}Y/^{64}Cu)-DOTA-ReCCMSH	Detection
	Ren et al[8]	^{18}F-SFB-RMSH-1	MC1 R expression
	Cantorias et al[10]	^{68}Ga-DOTA-ReCCMSH	Early diagnosis
Melanin Formation	van Langevelde[12]	^{11}C-l-dopa	Diagnosis
	Dimitrakopoulou-Strauss et al[14]	^{18}F-dopa	Metastasis
	Mishima et al[15]	^{18}F-^{10}B-L-BPA	Radiation planning
	van Ginkel et al[17]	L-[$^{1-11}$]C-tyrosine	Limb perfusion
Nicotinamide Analogues	Garg et al[18]	^{18}F-DAFBA	Tumor uptake
	Denoyer et al[20]	^{18}F-MEL050	Diagnosis
	Ren et al[21]	^{18}F-FBZA	Metastasis
Integrines	Beer et al[22]	^{18}F-galacto-RGD	Therapy
	Decristoforo et al[24]	^{68}Ga-DOTA-RGD	$\alpha_v\beta_3$ expression
	Wei et al[25]	^{64}Cu-CB-TE2A-c(RGDyK)	Angiogenesis
Reporter Gene Imaging	Shu et al[26]	^{18}F-FHBG	Therapy
	Brader et al[27]	^{18}F-FEAU PET	Lymph nodes status
Proliferation	Cobben et al[28]	^{18}F-FLT	Staging
	Ribas et al[29]	^{18}F-FLT	Lymph nodes status
	Solit et al[30]	^{18}F-FLT	Biologic response
Hypoxia Tracers	Wyss et al[32]	^{18}F-FMISO	Tumor uptake

Abbreviations: ^{18}F-^{10}B-L-BPA, ^{18}F-^{10}B-*p*-Boronophenylalanine; ^{18}F-DAFBA, N-(2-diethylaminoethyl)-4-^{18}F-fluorobenzamide; dopa, dihydroxyphenylalanine; FB, fluorobenzoate; FBZA; galacto-RGD; ^{18}F-Galacto-RGD, ^{18}F-Galacto-arginine-glycine-aspartic acid; ^{18}F-FEAU, ^{18}F-29-fluoro-29-deoxy-1-b-D-b-arabinofuranosyl-5-ethyluracil; ^{18}F-FBZA, N-[2-(diethylamino)-ethyl]-4-^{18}F-fluorobenzamide; ^{18}F-FLT, 3-^{18}F-fluoro-3-deoxy-L-thymidine; ^{18}F-FMISO, ^{18}F-fluoromisonidazole; MC1 R, melanocortin 1 receptor; MSH, Melanocyte-stimulating hormone.

developments in antibody engineering. Target antigens with high specificity are suitable candidates for tumor-specific targeting of PET radionuclides. Antibody fragments and engineered antibody derivatives, such as divalent, synthetic, single-chain Fv antibodies, have been constructed in an effort to accelerate clearance kinetics without a loss of tumor target specificity.[3] Voss and colleagues[4] presented data to demonstrate the feasibility of using sarcophagine chelator SarAr to produce stable immunoconjugates (labeled with copper 64), which are targets overexpressed in melanoma. The ^{64}Cu-SarAr monoclonal antibody system described in their study has a potential application in ^{64}Cu-PET imaging with a wide range of antibody- or peptide-based imaging agents.

MELANOCYTE-STIMULATING HORMONE ANALOGUES

One of the primary functions of α-melanocyte-stimulating hormone (α-MSH) is to regulate the biologic production of pigments in the skin, hair,

and eyes. Because this hormone binds to melanocortin 1 (MC1) receptors, which were found to be overexpressed in human melanoma cells, several peptide analogues of α-MSH have been synthesized for specific use in melanoma. However, nonspecific binding and a high accumulation in the kidney were seen in some of the analogues used, which would limit the potential clinical development of targeted melanoma agents because of possible nephrotoxicity. In an attempt to overcome this major problem, Froidevaux and colleagues[5] varied the position of DOTA conjugation, hydrophobicity, and the overall charge of a DOTA-α-MSH analogue labeled with gallium 68 to determine the effect on the retention in murine models of primary and metastatic melanoma, obtaining high-contrast images showing the clinical potential of this analogue in imaging.

Recently, Cheng and colleagues[6] evaluated the biodistribution of ^{64}Cu-DOTA-NAPamide in 2 mouse models to explore the potential use of the this agent in screening candidates for melanoma therapy. C57BL/6 mice bearing B16/F10 murine tumors (expressing a high density of MC1 receptors) and Fox Chase SCID mice bearing A375M human tumors (expressing a low density of MC1 receptors) were used to demonstrate that tumors with low MC1 receptor expression showed 50% less tumor uptake than those with higher MC1 expression. Furthermore, the accumulation of radioactivity was nonspecific only in the A375M tumors. This study underlines the need for further research on how pharmacokinetics of this particular melanoma-imaging agent can be improved.

A study by McQuade and colleagues[7] set out to label DOTA-ReCCMSH(Arg11) with β^+-emitting radionuclides using yttrium 86 and copper 64 complexes to determine if the high sensitivity of PET imaging could help detect malignant melanoma. Biodistribution and small animal PET imaging were performed in mice implanted with B16/F1 murine melanoma tumor and the results were compared with data obtained from the same animal model when using ^{18}F FDG. Both [86]Y and ^{64}Cu complexes reached a maximum tumor concentration at 30 minutes and small animal PET images confirmed that the tumor could be visualized after 30 minutes. These findings would suggest that DOTA-ReCCMSH(Arg11) labeled with β^+-emitting radionuclides has the potential for early detection of malignant melanoma because of the high sensitivity and resolution of PET. In a later study by Ren and colleagues,[8] the metallopeptide Ac-D-Lys-ReCCMSH(Arg11) was labeled with N-succinimidyl-4-^{18}F-fluorobenzoate (^{18}F-SFB). Both isomers of Ac-D-Lys-ReCCMSH(Arg11), named RMSH-1 and RMSH-2, were purified and identified by high-performance liquid chromatography. Both ^{18}F-labeled metallopeptides showed good tumor uptake in the B16/F10 murine model, with high MC1 receptor expression, but in the A375M human melanoma xenografted mice, the uptake was much lower, indicating a low MC1 receptor expression. Small animal PET of ^{18}F-SFB-RMSH-1 and 2 in B16/F10 tumor-bearing mice showed good tumor imaging quality. Therefore the radiofluorinated metallopeptide ^{18}F-FB-RMSH-1 seems to be a promising molecular probe for PET on tumors that are positive for MC1 receptor.

Wei and colleagues[9] described the synthesis and preclinical characterization of the MC1 receptor–targeting peptide CHX-A''-Re(Arg11)CCMSH in a study using B16/F1 melanoma-bearing mice labeled with yttrium 86 and gallium 68 demonstrating their ability to selectively target and image tumors in the B16/F1 mouse melanoma, suggesting their possible usefulness as melanoma-imaging agents in human patients. Cantorias and colleagues[10] reevaluated the tumor-targeting properties of high–specific activity ^{68}Ga-DOTA-Re(Arg11)CCMSH given to B16/F1 melanoma-bearing C57 mice. Bearing in mind that there are only a limited number of receptor sites in human and murine melanoma cell lines, purification was used to maximize specific activity. The production of high–specific activity ^{68}Ga-DOTA-Re(Arg11)CCMSH resulted in both greatly improved tumor uptake and tumor retention. The resulting PET images of the tumor showed a high degree of resolution because of the high tumor to non–target organ ratios at an early time point and the rapid elimination of the labeled peptide. The investigators suggest that high–specific activity ^{68}Ga-DOTA-Re(Arg11)CCMSH may have a future role in the early diagnosis of metastasized melanoma.

MELANIN FORMATION

Tyrosine is a well-known amino acid and is used for melanin formation. The amino acid is transported into the cells and transformed into dihydroxyphenylalanine (dopa). Some experimental data on the use of dopa in melanomas are already available. Ishiwata and colleagues[11] reported a high uptake of ^{18}F-dopa in experimental studies using rats that had received transplanted B18 melanoma cells. van Langevelde and colleagues[12] revealed for the first time the importance of l-dopa labeled with carbon 11 for diagnosing malignant melanoma on the basis of experimental data. Kubota and colleagues[13] showed that there was a preferential accumulation of ^{18}F-dopa in cells of the S phase in rats that had received transplanted B16 melanoma cells. Dimitrakopoulou-Strauss and colleagues[14] used ^{18}F-dopa in pretreated patients with metastatic melanoma in combination with [15O]water and FDG to gain more information about tumor biology. Their study aimed to explore the use of ^{18}F-dopa in detecting metastatic melanoma and to determine if the uptake was primarily an indicator of transport or metabolism of the radiopharmaceutical. The investigators suggest that ^{18}F-dopa can help identify viable melanoma metastases and thus may help in the selection of patients who could benefit from further treatment.

Diagnosis of human malignant melanoma by PET using [18]F-[10]B-p-Boronophenylalanine ([18]F-[10]B-L-BPA), a specific melanogenesis-seeking compound synthesized for use in boron neutron capture therapy (NCT) for melanoma, has been developed by Mishima and colleagues.[15] This development has resulted in a novel highly effective methodology for the selective 3-dimensional imaging of metastatic melanomas, and this methodology can also accurately determine the ^{10}B concentration in the tumor and surrounding tissues, providing almost all the diagnostic information needed for complete noninvasive radiation dose planning in the treatment of melanoma, both for NCT and for other types of therapy.

α-Aminoisobutyric acid (AIB) labeled with carbon 11 has been shown to be a useful imaging agent in patients with soft tissue cancers and melanoma, and it this agent has been used to demonstrate tumor uptake in a range of other animal tumor models. AIB is not metabolized after cellular uptake, and this property offers the possibility of studying amino acid transport into cells without interference because of radiolabeled metabolite formation. When used together with PET, AIB may permit the quantification of differences in amino acid transport between normal and malignant cells and act as a potential monitor of therapeutic intervention.[16] van Ginkel and colleagues[17] investigated PET with L-[^{1-11}C]tyrosine in patients with locally advanced soft tissue sarcoma and skin cancer of the lower limb who were undergoing hyperthermic isolated limb perfusion with recombinant tumor necrosis factor α and melphalan. PET gave a good indication of pathologic outcome, and viable tumor could be seen on the images without interference from posttreatment inflammatory tissue.

NICOTINAMIDE ANALOGUES

Clinical trials have shown that radiolabeled iodobenzamide derivates can be used to image cutaneous and ocular melanoma deposits with high specificity and sensitivity. In order to develop a PET radiopharmaceutical to image melanoma, Garg and colleagues[18] synthesized N-(2-diethylaminoethyl)-4-^{18}F-fluorobenzamide (^{18}F-DAFBA) and were able to demonstrate a rapid tumoral uptake of radioactivity in C57 mice bearing melanoma tumor xenograft. This result proved useful to delineate the tumor and its metastases in imaging applications. Greguric and colleagues[19] were able to construct a series of fluorine-based nicotinamide compounds that retained the attractive biologic properties displayed with radioiodinated iodobenzamide single-photon emission computed tomography analogues. It is already clear from these studies that ^{18}F-fluoronicotinamide will be a superior PET tracer for clinical staging because of its inherently higher lesion contrast. Compared with existing standards, including FDG, ^{18}F-fluoronicotinamide can offer a higher degree of sensitivity, especially in the detection of small metastases, and thereby allow more accurate selection and planning of treatment as well as better therapeutic monitoring in melanoma.

The most promising of these compounds seems to be MEL050, with its excellent tumor uptake, radiochemical stability, and pharmacokinetic properties, together with predominant renal excretion. Denoyer and colleagues[20] evaluated the melanoma-imaging potential of ^{18}F-MEL050 using PET and high-resolution autoradiography in murine models of primary and metastatic melanomas. They demonstrated that ^{18}F-MEL050 was capable of rapid tumor uptake and high retention, with specificity for melanin, which would indicate its great potential for noninvasive clinical evaluation of suspected melanoma. A recent publication by Ren and colleagues[21] describes the characterization of N-[2-(diethylamino)-ethyl]-4-^{18}F-fluorobenzamide (^{18}F-FBZA), a melanin-binding benzamide with a chemical structure similar to that of ^{18}F-MEL050. They found that ^{18}F-FBZA had lower tumor retention in B16 melanoma tumors than ^{18}F-MEL050. Furthermore, ^{18}F-FBZA appeared to be cleared partially through the hepatobiliary system, whereas there was no evidence of hepatic clearance for ^{18}F-MEL050. In addition, the radiosynthesis time for ^{18}F-FBZA was 3 hours compared with 1 hour for ^{18}F-MEL050. The investigators concluded that ^{18}F-MEL050 was a more likely candidate for use as a clinical PET tracer in melanoma imaging, especially for the identification of metastatic lesions in key organs, such as the liver and bowel. In this context, there is increasing interest in the use of novel molecular targeted therapies directed at key genes known to be associated with malignant melanoma.

INTEGRINS AND NEOANGIOGENESIS

Integrins are heterodimeric glycoproteins that are involved in cell-cell and cell-substratum interactions. One of these receptors is integrin $\alpha_v\beta_3$, which has been shown to play an essential role in the regulation of tumor growth, local invasiveness, and metastatic potential and is now under investigation as part of a strategy for anticancer therapy. Moreover, $\alpha_v\beta_3$ is also highly expressed on activated endothelial cells during angiogenesis. A study by Beer and colleagues[22] sets out to describe the biodistribution and pharmacokinetic behavior of ^{18}F-Galacto-arginine-glycine-aspartic acid (^{18}F-Galacto-RGD) in patients with cancer. Patients with melanomas and musculoskeletal sarcomas were chosen for this purpose because the role of $\alpha_v\beta_3$ in angiogenesis and metastatic potential had already been documented for these tumors. They found that ^{18}F-galacto-RGD allows a high-contrast visualization of $\alpha_v\beta_3$ expression in tumors. Consequently, this tracer offers a new strategy for the noninvasive monitoring of molecular processes, and the information that the tracer provides can be used in planning and controlling therapeutic approaches targeting the $\alpha_v\beta_3$ integrin. Another future avenue for research would be to document the $\alpha_v\beta_3$ expression of tumors before therapy with $\alpha_v\beta_3$ antagonists. ^{18}F-galacto-RGD could have a future clinical use in the noninvasive characterization of the biologic aggressiveness of a malignant tumor on an individual basis. Moreover, $\alpha_v\beta_3$ expression, confirmed noninvasively, might be used as a surrogate parameter of angiogenesis in those tumors that express this integrin only on endothelial cells and not on tumor cells.[23]

Decristoforo and colleagues[24] conducted a study that introduced ^{68}Ga-DOTA-RGD and compared its in vitro and in vivo properties with the corresponding ^{18}F-galacto-RGD. The greater ease of radiosynthesis of the former makes it seem an attractive alternative to monitor $\alpha_v\beta_3$ expression. Wei and colleagues[25] successfully synthesized and purified CB-TE2A-c(RGDyK) and diamsar-c(RGDfD) and radiolabeled both peptides with copper 64. The concentration in melanoma of ^{64}Cu-CB-TE2A-c(RGDyK) in the $\alpha_v\beta_3$-positive M21 tumor was found to be higher than that of the negative control M21L tumor. The $\alpha_v\beta_3$ binding affinities of the 2 Cu-chelator-RGD peptides were similar. Of the 2 peptides, ^{64}Cu-CB-TE2A-c (RGDyK) is a superior compound for $\alpha_v\beta_3$ integrin targeting because it provides a higher degree of tumor uptake, faster liver and blood clearance, and a higher tumor/blood ratio. Both ^{64}Cu-CB-TE2A-c(RGDyK) and ^{64}Cu-diamsar-c(RGDfD) are potential candidates for imaging tumor angiogenesis.

OTHER APPROACHES

In patients with melanoma, the outlook is determined by regional lymph node status. Current imaging modalities are limited in their ability to detect micrometastases in lymph nodes, and a more sensitive technique is needed to accurately identify occult lymph node metastases. PET-based reporter gene imaging is a growing field to allow monitoring cancer therapy. Shu and colleagues[26] enabled detection of T cells after adoptive transfer with the PET reporter gene *sr39tk* labeled with 9-[4-[^{18}F]fluoro-3-(hydroxy-methyl)-butyl]guanine (^{18}F-FHBG), suggesting a significant clinical utility for providing early predictions of treatment efficacy. A second study by Brader and colleagues[27] was to develop a noninvasive method for the detection of micrometastases in regional lymph nodes using a replication-competent oncolytic virus. Their results show, for the first time, that oncolytic viruses introduced into the lymphatic system via a single intratumoral injection can reliably detect melanoma micrometastases in regional lymph nodes using ^{18}F FFAU PET imaging. This murine model needs to be studied in clinical trials to verify if it can improve the staging and management of patients with melanoma.

Cobben and colleagues[28] investigated the utility of 3-^{18}F-fluoro-3-deoxy-L-thymidine (^{18}F-FLT) PET for staging patients with clinical stage III melanoma. The series had only 10 patients and no comparisons with ^{18}F FDG-PET were made, so valid conclusions on the potential role of this radiotracer cannot be drawn purely on the basis of their results. Nevertheless, in 3 patients, ^{18}F FLT PET detected a total of 3 additional lesions that had therapeutic consequences but without changing the staging. These lesions had been missed by the initial clinical staging. There are 2 studies that analyze the role of ^{18}F FLT PET in the assessment of melanoma treatment response. Ribas and colleagues[29] tested the role of whole body molecular imaging in patients with advanced melanoma who were receiving the CTLA4-blocking antibody tremelimumab, with the PET probe ^{18}F-FDG being used for the analysis of changes in glucose metabolism, and ^{18}F-FLT, for cell replication changes. ^{18}F-FLT allows the mapping and noninvasive imaging of cell proliferation in secondary lymphoid organs after CTLA4 blockade in patients with melanoma. A second study by Solit and colleagues[30] suggested that ^{18}F FLT PET can effectively detect the induction of gap 1 (G_1) phase arrest by mitogen-activated protein kinase/extracellular signal-regulated kinase kinase (MEK) inhibitors in mutant BRAF melanoma tumors and may be a useful noninvasive method for the assessment of early biologic response to this family of drugs.

An important characteristic of malignant tumors is that they are often poorly perfused and have areas of low oxygenation. Such hypoxic regions can prove resistant to standard external beam radiation therapy and some forms of chemotherapy. Identifying hypoxic cells in vivo is important in management terms because they are less responsive to both radiation therapy and chemotherapy. Hypoxia has varying effects on metabolic tracers used for PET. Clavo and Wahl[31] reported that in vitro exposure of tumor cells to 4 hours of hypoxia decreased tumor uptake of thymidine (a marker of DNA synthesis) in 2 different malignant human tumor cell lines, including melanoma, but increased FDG uptake in both lines. Levels of L-leucine (a marker of protein synthesis) uptake declined in both cell lines with moderate hypoxia, which was consistent with reduced protein synthesis. Over this period of hypoxia methionine uptake was not significantly changed in either cell line. Based on these in vitro observations, it is probable that oxygen concentrations in local tissue can affect the metabolic signals observed using PET in in vivo human tumors. Paired hypoxia-sensitive PET tracers have a potential use for noninvasive characterization of tissue oxygenation levels. Wyss and colleagues[32] tried to assess the potential and utility of ultrahigh resolution hypoxia imaging in their study of various murine tumor models using the established hypoxia PET tracer ^{18}F-fluoromisonidazole (^{18}F-FMISO). In 10 of 11 experimental tumor models including B16 melanoma, ^{18}F FMISO PET imaging provided clear-cut visualization of the tumors.

In conclusion, in the search for improvement, the current literature on melanoma management using radiotracers other than FDG is still quite limited, and most works published to date are preclinical studies. However, on the whole, results reported so far are promising, especially in the development of highly specific agents which will probably lead to an earlier and more precise diagnosis and to a patient-by-patient treatment, which will have a significant effect on the management of patients with melanoma.

SUMMARY

[18]F FDG-PET has proven its use as a technique in the field of melanoma, but there are valid concerns related to the specificity of ^{18}F FDG-PET findings and the degree of accuracy we can expect in the assessment of response to new treatment protocols. The main avenues currently being explored for future use in staging and management of melanoma with PET other than FDG include monoclonal antibodies against melanoma-associated antigens, α-MSH analogues, amino acids involved in melanin formation, nicotinamide-based compounds, heterodimeric glycoproteins such as integrins, reporter gene imaging, cell proliferation, and hypoxia tracers.

REFERENCES

1. Avril NE, Weber WA. Monitoring response to treatment in patients utilizing PET. Radiol Clin North Am 2005;43(1):189–204.
2. Eisenhauer EA, Therasse P, Bogaerts J, et al. New response evaluation criteria in solid tumours: revised RECIST guideline (version 1.1). Eur J Cancer 2009; 45(2):228–47.
3. Wu AM, Senter PD. Arming antibodies: prospects and challenges for immunoconjugates. Nat Biotechnol 2005;23(9):1137–46.
4. Voss SD, Smith SV, DiBartolo N, et al. Positron emission tomography (PET) imaging of neuroblastoma and melanoma with 64Cu-SarAr immunoconjugates. Proc Natl Acad Sci 2007;104(44):17489–93.
5. Froidevaux S, Calame-Christe M, Tanner H, et al. Melanoma targeting with DOTA-α-melanocyte-stimulating hormone analogs: structural parameters affecting tumor uptake and kidney uptake. J Nucl Med 2005;46(5):887–95.
6. Cheng Z, Xiong Z, Subbarayan M, et al. 64Cu-labeled alpha-melanocyte-stimulating hormone for microPET imaging of melanocortin 1 receptor expression. Bioconjug Chem 2007;18(3):765–72.
7. McQuade P, Miao Y, Yoo J, et al. Imaging of melanoma using 64Cu- and 86Y-DOTA-ReCCMSH (Arg11), a cyclized peptide analogue of r-MSH. J Med Chem 2005;48(8):2985–92.
8. Ren G, Liu Z, Miao Z, et al. PET of Malignant melanoma using 18F-labeled metallopeptides. J Nucl Med 2009;50(11):1865–72.
9. Wei L, Zhang X, Gallazzi F, et al. Melanoma imaging using 111In-, 86Y- and 68Ga-labeled CHX-A″-Re (Arg11)CCMSH. Nucl Med Biol 2009;36(4):345–54.
10. Cantorias MV, Figueroa SD, Quinn TP, et al. Development of high-specific-activity 68Ga-labeled DOTA-rhenium-cyclized α-MSH peptide analog to target MC1 receptors overexpressed by melanoma tumors. Nucl Med Biol 2009;36(5):505–13.
11. Ishiwata K, Kubota K, Kubota R, et al. Selective 2-(F-18) fluorodopa uptake for melanogenesis in murine metastatic melanomas. J Nucl Med 1991;32(1):95–101.
12. van Langevelde A, van der Molen HD, Journée-de Korver JG, et al. Potential radiopharmaceuticals for the detection of ocular melanoma. Part III. A study with 14C and 11C labelled tyrosine and dihydroxyphenylalanine. Eur J Nucl Med 1988;14(7):382–7.
13. Kubota R, Yamada S, Ishiwata K, et al. Active melanogenesis in non-S phase melanocytes in B16 melanomas in vivo investigated by double-tracer microautoradiography with 18F-fluorodopa and 3H-thymidine. Br J Cancer 1992;66(4):614–8.
14. Dimitrakopoulou-Strauss A, Strauss LG, Burger C. Quantitative PET studies in pretreated melanoma patients: a comparison of 6-[18F] fluoro-L-dopa with 18F-FDG and 15O-water using compartment and noncompartment analysis. J Nucl Med 2001; 42(2):248–56.
15. Mishima Y, Imahori Y, Honda C, et al. In vivo diagnosis of human malignant melanoma with positron emission tomography using specific melanoma-seeking 18F-DOPA analogue. J Neurooncol 1997;33(1):163–9.
16. Schmall B, Conti PS, Alauddin MM. Synthesis of [11C-methyl]-alpha-aminoisobutyric acid (AIB). Nucl Med Biol 1996;23(3):263–6.
17. van Ginkel RJ, Kole AC, Nieweg OE, et al. L-[1-11C]-tyrosine PET to evaluate response to hyperthermic isolated limb perfusion for locally advanced soft-

tissue sarcoma and skin cancer. J Nucl Med 1999; 40(2):262–7.

18. Garg S, Kothari K, Thopate SR, et al. Design, synthesis, and preliminary in vitro and in vivo evaluation of N-(2-diethylaminoethyl)-4-[18F]fluorobenzamide ([18F]-DAFBA): a novel potential PET probe to image melanoma tumors. Bioconjug Chem 2009;20(3):583–90.

19. Greguric I, Taylor SR, Denoyer D, et al. Discovery of [18F]N-(2-(diethylamino) ethyl)-6-fluoronicotinamide: a melanoma positron emission tomography imaging radiotracer with high tumor to body contrast ratio and rapid renal clearance. J Med Chem 2009; 52(17):5299–302.

20. Denoyer D, Greguric I, Roselt P, et al. High-contrast PET of melanoma using 18F-MEL050, a selective probe for melanin with predominantly renal clearance. J Nucl Med 2010;51(3):441–7.

21. Ren G, Miao Z, Liu H, et al. Melanin-targeted preclinical PET imaging of melanoma metastasis. J Nucl Med 2009;50(10):1692–9.

22. Beer AJ, Haubner R, Goebel M, et al. Biodistribution and pharmacokinetics of the $\alpha_v\beta_3$-selective tracer 18F-galacto-RGD in cancer patients. J Nucl Med 2005;46(8):1333–41.

23. Beer AJ, Haubner R, Wolf I, et al. PET-based human dosimetry of 18F-galacto-RGD, a new radiotracer for imaging $\alpha_v\beta_3$ expression. J Nucl Med 2006;47(5): 763–9.

24. Decristoforo C, Hernandez Gonzalez I, Carlsen J, et al. 68Ga- and 111In-labelled DOTA-RGD peptides for imaging of $\alpha v\beta 3$ integrin expression. Eur J Nucl Med Mol Imaging 2008;35(8):1507–15.

25. Wei L, Yea Y, Thaddeus J, et al. 64Cu-Labeled CB-TE2A and diamsar-conjugated RGD peptide analogs for targeting angiogenesis: comparison of their biological activity. Nucl Med Biol 2009;36(3): 277–85.

26. Shu CJ, Radu CG, Shelly SM, et al. Quantitative PET reporter gene imaging of CD8+ T cells specific for a melanoma-expressed self-antigen. Int Immunol 2009;21(2):155–65.

27. Brader P, Kelly K, Gang S, et al. Imaging of lymph node micrometastases using an oncolytic herpes virus and [18F]FEAU PET. PLoS One 2009;4(3):e4789.

28. Cobben DCP, Jager PL, Elsinga PH, et al. 3-18F-Fluoro-3-Deoxy-L-thymidine: a new tracer for staging metastatic melanoma? J Nucl Med 2003;44(12): 1927–32.

29. Ribas A, Benz MR, Allen-Auerbach MS, et al. Imaging of CTLA4 blockade–induced cell replication with 18F-FLT PET in patients with advanced melanoma treated with tremelimumab. J Nucl Med 2010;51(3):340–6.

30. Solit DB, Santos E, Pratilas CA, et al. 3′-Deoxy-3′-[18F] fluorothymidine positron emission tomography is a sensitive method for imaging the response of BRAF-dependent tumors to MEK inhibition. Cancer Res 2007;67(23):11463–9.

31. Clavo AC, Wahl RL. Effects of hypoxia on the uptake of tritiated thymidine, L-leucine, L-methionine and FDG in cultured cancer cells. J Nucl Med 1996;37(3):502–6.

32. Wyss MT, Honer M, Schubiger PA, et al. NanoPET imaging of [18F]fluoromisonidazole uptake in experimental mouse tumours. Eur J Nucl Med Mol Imaging 2006;33(3):311–8.

Index

Note: Page numbers of article titles are in **boldface** type.

A

α-Aminobutyric acid, carbon-labeled, 94
ABCD(E)s, of melanoma, 2
Acral-lentiginous melanoma, 3
Adrenal glands, metastasis to, structural
    imaging for, 44
Advanced melanoma
    PET/CT for, **27–35**
    structural imaging for, **37–54**
Age, melanoma prognosis and, 19
Amelanotic melanoma, 3
American Joint Committee on Cancer TNM
    classification, 3–5, 28–29
Angiography, for ocular melanoma, 81
Animal studies, PET for, **71–77**
Anorectal melanoma, 85
Antibodies, monoclonal, against
    melanoma-associated antigens, 91–92
Asymmetry, of lesions, 2
Axilla, sentinel nodes in, 15

B

Benzamide compounds, 74–75
Biliary tract, metastasis to, structural
    imaging for, 39–43
Biopsy, 2, 5. *See also* Sentinel node biopsy.
    fine-needle aspiration
        for recurrent melanoma, 65
        ultrasound with, 19–20
Bladder, metastasis to, structural imaging for, 44–46
Bleeding, 2
Blue dye, for intraoperative sentinel node detection,
    17–18
Bone, metastasis to
    CT for, 28
    MR imaging for, 28
    structural imaging for, 49–50
Bone marrow, metastasis to, structural
    imaging for, 49–50
Borders, of lesions, 2
Boron neutron capture therapy, 93–94
Brachytherapy, for ocular melanoma, 83
Brain
    melanoma of, 86
    metastasis to, 60
        MR imaging for, 28
        PET/CT for, 32
Breslow depth, 4, 29

C

CCMSH compounds, 72, 93
CDKB2A gene, mutations in, 2
Cervical nodes, 15
Chemotherapy
    for head and neck melanoma, 85
    response to, PET/CT for, 31–32
Choroid, melanoma of, 80–83
Ciliary body, melanoma of, 80
Clark level, 4–5
Collaborative Ocular Melanoma Study group, 81
Color, of lesions, 2
Completion lymph node dissection, 10–12
Computed tomography. *See* CT.
Conjunctiva, melanoma of, 80
Contrast agents, for MR imaging, 38–39
Contrast-enhanced CT, for advanced
    melanoma, 28, 30
Copper 64 compounds, 92–93
CT. *See also* PET/CT.
    for adrenal metastasis, 44
    for advanced melanoma, 28, **37–54**
    for biliary tract metastasis, 39–43
    for bladder metastasis, 44–46
    for bone and bone marrow metastasis, 49–50
    for gallbladder metastasis, 39–43
    for gastrointestinal metastasis, 46–47
    for heart metastasis, 48–49
    for kidney metastasis, 44–46
    for liver metastasis, 39–43
    for lung metastasis, 48–49
    for lymph node metastasis, 47–48
    for mesentery metastasis, 47–48
    for ocular melanoma, 81–82
    for pancreas metastasis, 43–44
    for recurrent melanoma, 59–66
    for soft tissue metastasis, 49, 51
    for spleen metastasis, 43
    for ureter metastasis, 44–46
    usefulness of, 37–39
    whole-body, 44

D

[^{18}F]-DAFBA (N-(2-diethylaminoethyl)-4-[^{18}F]-
    fluorobenzamide), 94
Desmoplastic melanoma, 3
Diameter, of lesions, 2

PET Clin 6 (2011) 99–103
doi:10.1016/S1556-8598(11)00024-1

Printed and bound by CPI Group (UK) Ltd, Croydon, CR0 4YY

03/10/2024

01040350-0015